ANXIETY

Understand How Neuroscience and the Universe Works Together to Stop Overthinking. Rewire your Brain Using Vagus Nerve Power to Overcome Anxiety, Panic Attacks, Fear, Worry and Shyness

By
Maria Carter

Table Of Contents
ASTROLOGY

Table Of Contents
VAGUS NERVE

ASTROLOGY

A Beginners Guide To Horoscopes And The 12 Zodiac Signs To Master Your Destiny And Spiritual Growth. Finding Yourself And Others Through Numerology And Kundalini Rising

(SOUL PURPOSE)

By
Maria Carter

Introduction To Astrology And Celestial Influences

Congratulations on downloading *"Astrology: A Beginners Guide to Understand Yourself and Others through the 12 Zodiac Signs and Horoscopes for Spiritual Growth. Master your Destiny thanks to Numerology and Kundalini Rising (Empath)"* and thank you for doing so.

The significance of astrology is still notable to numerous societies. The individuals of India and China put incredible confidence in soothsaying even today. They practice the craft of soothsaying in their daily lives and base significant choices on the science.

In this cutting edge time of innovation and science with heterodox contemplations and ideas, do you think crystal gazing is huge? Soothsaying is an old idea, as old as time, you can say. It is a significant part of our lives – our past, present, and future. As it were, crystal gazing is utilized to conjecture and anticipate future occasions and can likewise be utilized as a medium to dispose of any sort of disaster identified with planetary positions.

The idea that planetary bodies in the close planetary system can really give a dream of things to come has intrigued individuals for quite a while. Our inclinations with soothsaying range from a standard look at a paper's zodiac signs area to settling on noteworthy choices in life- identified with marriage, fund and vocation and even expectations on wellbeing. It is realized that numerous effective individuals have counseled celestial prophets to help settle on choices in their lives.

One part of crystal gazing is that it influences our lives. The various developments of the moon or the planetary developments or arrangements influence our psyches and feelings and we don't understand this. The planetary situations at the hour of our introduction to the world in the prophetic graph can be contrasted and the planetary situation of whenever. This investigation will indicate how a specific planet or two impact our lives, as it were, at a given time. The outcome might be certain or negative, yet these correlations feature the adjustment in our lives or our states of mind and responses to occasions. This is only crystal gazing.

The planetary developments have their effect on us, however, we are likewise influenced by the planetary developments of the individuals whom we manage, be it our folks, companion, kids, relatives, companions, associates, supervisors, colleagues, and so on. These individuals are likewise influenced by soothsaying as much as we may be.

Chapter 1

Getting To Know The 12 House Systems

It is important to acknowledge the fact that those who wish to study Astrology should put themselves in a situation where all inputs provided to them should be accepted wholly. There shouldn't be any doubts or negativities as these energies can greatly affect the representation of the stars. Moreover, this book will also address any misconceptions an individual may have on certain astrological points. Nevertheless, do keep in mind that this book will focus on one's road to understanding themselves by reading their astrological alignment. With this in mind, let's begin with the very basic fundamental of them all – the house systems.

In Astrology, houses speak to an approach to make each minute in time close to home and brought down to the degree of planet Earth. They are an outcome of our planet's pivot and come to presence by division of the ecliptic plane into twelve pieces. In Western Astrology, there are a few house frameworks that are as yet utilized, while the most well-known one right now is the Placidus framework.

In one day, an Ascendant (first house cusp) will travel through the majority of the signs in the zodiacal circle. An Ascendant and a Descendant in every natal graph get characterized before breakfast and nightfall, or minutes when the Sun is ascending in the East and setting in the West. This is the reason an individual will have the Sun close to their Ascendant in the event that they are conceived at day break and close to their Descendant on the off chance that they are conceived at twilight. When all is said in done, the Sun will be over the skyline and in one of the upper houses on the off chance that you were conceived by daytime, and the Sun beneath the skyline on the off chance that you were conceived at evening time. Houses are numbered counterclockwise from the cusp of the principal house and constantly anticipated on the ecliptic.

In the event that you envision yourself in your natal graph, you will see that above you are the planets over the skyline. In the event that you have to feel an association with the Universe you can see, turn upward in the sky around evening time, and you will consider them to be indistinguishable situations from they remain in the outline existing apart from everything else. The main distinction here is in their direction, since the outline drawing contrasts from our typical idea of the East and the West, putting East on the left and West on the right. Tragically, you won't have the option to see the houses since they are anecdotal lines used to separate the hover into twelve pieces.

We can utilize space or time as a reason for the division of houses. They are constantly numbered counterclockwise from the cusp of the primary house, and this cusp (the Ascendant) will be characterized by the eastern point at a particular minute. In the event that our division depends on space, the plane is partitioned into equivalent circular segments of 30° each. On the off chance that the premise is time, houses are either invariant, and speak to 2 hours of the Sun's evident development each, or fleeting, when daytime and evening time are partitioned into six equivalent parts.

Whatever their division, we are constantly mindful that a whole graph has 360 degrees. The significant thing to recall however lies in the way that all frameworks will bode well up to some point. The Placidus framework has demonstrated to be genuinely huge, as the pioneer in its utilization, yet this doesn't imply that you shouldn't evaluate different frameworks as well, and check whether you coexist better with a portion of the others.

The Equal House Systems

The sign-house framework is one of the most streamlined frameworks of houses still being used. Here, the Ascendant is viewed as just to characterize the rising sign and the primary house starts at this current sign's zero degrees. Each after sign compares to the accompanying house until the circle is finished. This framework was the fundamental framework in the Hellenistic custom of Astrology is still being used in Vedic Astrology.

The equivalent house framework likewise partitions the ecliptic into twelve bits of 30 degrees, however the principal house cusp is characterized by the Ascendant or the eastern purpose of dawn. This framework is for the most part utilized today in higher scopes, particularly over 60 degrees, where the Placidean framework is very misshaped. In both of these frameworks, Midheaven or the most elevated point in the outline (MC) doesn't speak to a tenth house cusp. Rather, it moves around any of the houses over the skyline.

The Quadrant House Systems

Quadrant house frameworks partition the houses by four points – Ascendant, Nadir (Imum Coeli), Descendant and Midheaven (Medium Coeli). We consider them the edges of every horoscope as they speak to emphatically complemented houses where each planet gets exceptional quality of impact in an individual's life. We will just make reference to some of them here, pertinent for our work here, or normally utilized in various visionary methodologies today.

Porphyry's and Regiomontanus

The least complex quadrant house framework is Porphyry's framework, which partitions every quadrant of the ecliptic into three equivalent parts. It speaks to the base for all other quadrant house frameworks in spite of the fact that their definite focuses are determined in an unexpected way. In the event that the heavenly equator is isolated into twelve, and these divisions anticipated on the ecliptic, we get the Regiomontanus framework. It is for the most part out of utilization as of now, yet it was a significant antecedent of the most regularly utilized framework in present-day Western Astrology – Placidus arrangement of houses.

The Placidus House System

The Placidus house framework depends on every level of the ecliptic moving from nadir to the skyline, and from the skyline to the Midheaven. The fundamental issue this framework needs to face is in higher scopes, in light of the fact that specific degrees never contact the skyline and planets falling in them can't be doled out into houses without expanding the framework. In the event that you make a graph for some far off northern city, you will see that the twisting "swallows" the diagram and makes is difficult to utilize houses by any means, when the sum total of what you have are two enormous houses, and those remaining beside them.

The Meridian House System

Despite the fact that there are other house frameworks that were significant at some crossroads ever, these are the ones that will be important for our work. This rundown wouldn't be finished without a really uncommon substance – Meridian house framework, which partitions the divine equator into twelve bits of 30 degrees and activities them to the ecliptic along the extraordinary circles containing the North and the South heavenly shafts. In spite of the fact that you will likely once in a while use it, this house framework can really prove to be useful in migration crystal gazing.

House Modalities

Much the same as indications of the zodiac have their quality/methodology and have a place with a specific component of Nature, houses have comparative methods for articulation. Precise houses are those characterized by beginning stages of quadrants, which means they are at horoscope's points – first, fourth, seventh and tenth house. These houses speak to action and the vitality to push ahead and are in a manner associated with the idea of Mars. Succedent houses are those that pursue precise ones, shielded from every one of the progressions and an excessive amount of development. They are firmly associated with soundness, helping us to remember a ton of the fixed sign quality. These houses are second, fifth, eighth and eleventh. Cadent houses are third, sixth, ninth and twelfth and they are somewhat dubious, for they appear to be forerunners to what comes in the following precise house. These are houses associated principally to the way toward adapting, yet we shouldn't disregard their job as a reason for anything made by exercises done later on in rakish houses.

The Four Elements: Fire, Earth, Air, and Water

Like zodiac signs, houses likewise have a place with the four components of nature. Much the same as their relating signs, every one of them conveys a story in its component. This for all intents and purposes implies that the main house compares with the indication of Aries, and accordingly – has a place with the component of Fire. The equivalent goes for each house that pursues – the subsequent house having a place with the component of Earth, the third to Air, the fourth to Water, and so forth.

Visionary Interpretations

Each house is one's natal diagram, or any outline so far as that is concerned, speaks to the closest to home and natural device to be utilized in any examination. The house itself speaks to a spot or a territory wherein a planet is situated in. For instance, the fourth house will discuss numerous things, yet most truly, it will portray a home of an individual and what's in it. With Venus here, for instance, we will see delightful things, adornments, cash or a darling holding up at home.

It is essential to recall that much of the time, the planet will talk about a particular individual or thing that the vitality is centered around, the sign will give a shut portrayal of the planet, and the house will discuss area regarding an everyday issue wherein the planet will appear or show. The principal house is in a manner an exemption to this standard since it talks legitimately to the physical body of the individual being referred to. Be that as it may, regardless it stays attached to the component of Earth as it were, way more close to home than all else, and for the most part dispassionate and concrete.

The Ruler

Houses have cusps in various indications of the zodiac, and this gives them a stretch of an arm to be moreover translated through their ruler. The house is decided by the planet that principles the sign it falls into. So to explain, if the third house falls in the indication of Virgo, which means its cusp is in this sign, the house's ruler will be the leader of Virgo - Mercury.

It isn't in every case simple to characterize the significance of the house ruler contrasting with the idea of the planet itself and the idea of the sign it rules. This is the reason the best activity is to remember that precise houses show firmly and their rulers speak to defining moments throughout everybody's life. Each and every other elucidation will be, such as everything, a moderate and adjusted methodology that thinks about all elements in the perfect sum.

In spite of the fact that our horoscope diagram is two dimensional (level), the segments of the houses are most certainly not. They are three dimensional, similarly as the areas of an orange seem to be. Envision strolling outside under the night sky, with the stars and planets twinkling around you, and after that envision splitting the majority of that space, the space above and underneath you (on the opposite side of the earth) into twelve segments or portions. From where you stand, looking toward the south would be the tenth House, behind you and toward the north (and beneath you) would be the fourth House, at your left and toward the east would be the First House, on your right side and toward the west would be the seventh House, etc. This is the thing that celestial houses are.

House Cusps

House cusps are controlled by taking the 3-dimensional house segments (recall the portions of an orange) and seeing where these lines meet and cross the zodiac. Where these lines cross the zodiac is the cusp for each house, and the zodiac sign there is said to be the "sign on the house cusp." In the chart above, you can see the house sections, and you can likewise observe the ring of the twelve zodiac signs. Where each section cuts over the band of the zodiac is the place a sign is on a house cusp. Albeit most house frameworks are partitioned into the recognizable twelve houses, there is a wide range of sorts of house frameworks; that is, there are numerous marginally various methods for splitting the space that encompasses us. Soothsayers like to contend among themselves with respect to which house framework is the best, and they consent to vary on this.

The Meaning of the Twelve Houses

Every one of the twelve houses has an alternate importance, and each portrays or calls attention to an alternate region of our experience. When we pick up something about what every one of these territories of experience implies, we can start perusing visionary sentences like the one given above, "Sun in Cancer in the Eighth House." And, the best part is that the wheel of the twelve houses is, itself, a brought together, entire cycle (just like the zodiac signs, the periods of the Moon, and so on.), with the goal that each house in the cycle is a stage, one prompting the following; consequently, when you find out about cycles and cycles' stages, you are naturally finding out about the houses.

First House

In each close to home elucidation, the principal house characterizes an individual, their physical body, qualities, and shortcomings, just like their base character. It is additionally named The House of Self, talking about our principle task throughout everyday life, our viewpoint into the world, conscience, and all that we are here to begin. It is our base vitality, associates us to the indication of Aries and our first chakra, and talks about the potential we have to suffer through any close to home fights or manners by which we can maintain a strategic distance from them. Its Latin maxim is Vita, making it "the place of Life itself".

The principal house is the fundamental association we have to our body and the manifestation we are in right now. This is actually why it is the most significant window into our universe of karmic obligation and speaks to the degree of straightforwardness or hardship we need to experience so as to develop in this lifetime. On the off chance that one has a test seen through planets set in the main house or its ruler, it ends up evident that they have an errand to determine and an obligation to reimburse while in this body. Every positive viewpoint, or a planet in its solid nobility, will talk about endowments we have assembled in past lifetimes or through our family tree, whatever your picked point of view.

The First House in Aries

On the off chance that your Ascendant is set in the indication of Aries, regardless of in the event that it falls on its first or last degree, it makes you an Arian. This position talks about the significance of knowing one's confines, essential instinctual vitality, and carnal nature that should be guided, utilized, and in some cases contained. The principle challenge of this position lies in the failure to consider others to be as equivalents, have civility, care for other people or acknowledge being thought about. It will provoke one's responsibility to connections, marriage or their capacity to discover empathy for their very own enthusiastic needs, not to mention the requirements of other individuals. On an individual level, these individuals are spoken to via planet Mars.

The First House in Taurus

On the off chance that an individual diagram starts in Taurus, we see an individual of natural delights, looking for adoration, indulgence, and fulfillment. Contingent upon the degree of difficulties this sign, house or Venus have, it tends to be a fine position that enables us to appreciate life in full shading and utilizing the majority of our faculties. This talks about an individual well-constructed, solid and static, and furthermore somewhat aloof. With an Ascendant in Taurus, you may be inclined to put on weight or pursue such a large number of delights through reckless conduct. The best challenge for a Taurus is to acknowledge the need and the magnificence of progress. When remembered, it can free these people to indicate activity, energy, and when required – the battle for their fulfillment. This is somebody spoken to by Venus.

The First House in Gemini

In the event that one is to begin their life in the body of a Gemini, they need to consistently remain to progress. This is an indication of verbally expressed word, insight, fast encounters, change of character, and development of numerous types. Individuals brought into the world with this rising sign are regularly quick, meager, mobile, insecure, and at times shallow. They have to remain well-educated, invaded in their social condition, and consistently have the motivation to convey or conceptualize issues that encompass them day by day. Their most prominent test is to concentrate on one objective, a point in reality that gives their life reason. They have to discover an amalgamation, one thing to cover the majority of their data and structure an accomplished supposition simply in the wake of learning their inward truth. They are spoken to by Mercury.

The First House in Cancer

At the point when the principal house starts in the indication of Cancer, it is frequently said to be the indication of home, family, and feeling. What we regularly neglect to comprehend is the affectability of this sign and its impact on our physical body. The ascendant speaks to our physical quality and this isn't the most ideal situation to feel solid and sure or to exercise, or train. Malignant growth people are regularly pale, unequivocally impacted by the developments of the Moon, tend to resemble the nourishment they eat, and consistently affect their general wellbeing and appearance. Their most noteworthy test is covered up in solid plans, relentless will, a sound daily practice, and obligation they need to take for the course their very own life is moving in. This is a sign administered by the Moon.

The First House in Leo

With your first house set in the indication of Leo, there is constantly a personality fight that must be perceived. This is a red hot sign that enables these individuals' valiance and to show themselves in the most ideal light in the most testing of circumstances. They are gone to themselves, with a solid physical make-up however little desire to invest an excess of energy working. Warm and cuddly, those brought into the world with the rising indication of Leo can be staggeringly "delicate around the edges", with huge, round ears, attractive, and wearing new and marked garments. Their most prominent test is to liberate the image they make out of vanity. They have to perceive their distinction and don't hesitate to stick out, be extraordinary, turned into a revolutionary and consider the prosperity of mankind. Their ruler is the King of the skies – the Sun.

The First House in Virgo

On the off chance that your ascendant fell in the indication of Virgo, this could undoubtedly be a sign that you were destined to help other people. Despite the fact that this is the sign wherein Mercury is lifted up, it doesn't invigorate a lot to one's physical constitution and talks about a wide range of medical problems that may surface. It is an indication that demonstrates a fine constitution, somebody who resembles a library type, with glasses, flimsy hear and a solid conviction framework with regards to all issues of mending. In addition to this, it will discuss insight and mental clearness. The greatest test of these people is to see the master plan, separate from dull subtleties and have some confidence in the more prominent request of things. This prompts their issues with trust and makes them powerless against a wide range of misdirection. Their ruler is Mercury.

The First House in Libra

In the event that your first house cusp is set in the indication of Libra, it resembles your entire horoscope is flipped around. While one ought to have the option to empty the vitality from Self, individuals brought into the world with this Ascendant need to discover it in individuals they are encompassed with, consistently looking for parity, and discovering approaches to retouch connections to the point in which they don't trigger weariness. This will make an individual that should be sharp looking and respectful consistently, frequently neglecting to go to physical exercises and individual limits in connection to other people. The best challenge a Libra's first house needs to defeat is the acknowledgment of displeasure and useful clash. They are spoken to by Venus.

The First House in Scorpio

To be brought into the world with an Ascendant in the indication of Scorpio, one must have a mind-blowing association with the material world. This is somebody solid, fixed and decided, yet additionally profoundly touchy and passionate, anyway hard these people may attempt to oppose this reality. This is an indication of dull cosmetics, individuals with solid, dim hair, enormous noses, and savage mentality continually shining from their profound eyes. Regardless of whether they are brought into the world fair, the look in their eyes will consistently demonstrate the power inside, as though they needed to defeat passing even before they were conceived. The enormous test here is to acknowledge the excellence of consistent fulfillment, feel appreciation and excuse the individuals who brought hurt or agony into their lives. Fault, possessive and over the top conduct are only a portion of the signs that they experience difficulty acknowledging what keeps them solid and alive. They are managed by Mars and Pluto.

The First House in Sagittarius

Those brought into the world with the Ascendant in Sagittarius frequently get the opportunity to be physically bigger than other individuals in their family tree. If not, their point of view gets the chance to be more extensive, their feelings solid and their psyches critical. Savants and instructors, these people can see the master plan, yet regularly experience difficulty remaining reasonable, while battling with their need to see the world through pink goggles. Continually looking forward, they are generally fun and a delight to be with. The test they need to face covers up in their nonsensical methodology. They have an undertaking to perceive keen, sensible and down to earth sides to everything in their life. This is a sign administered by helpful Jupiter.

The First House in Capricorn

On the off chance that somebody's Ascendant is set in the indication of Capricorn, they will be reasonable and gone to material issues and objectives in life they believe they need to accomplish. Contingent upon the places of planets in this house and its ruler, they will be fruitful or tested in their span for a specific goal, characterizing whether they will have the option to make an arrangement they can pursue. This can be an indication that talks about a substantial cross that should be conveyed, similarly as it can discuss a down to earth individual ready to perceive the utilization in everything that occurs in their life. Solid and firm, these individuals regularly have a fit to take care of, issues with their spine and bones, or their confidence in God and their connection to religion. Their greatest test is to discover comprehension and empathy for those that are powerless, excessively delicate or firmly enthusiastic. Their ruler is Saturn.

The First House in Aquarius

With an Ascendant in Aquarius, no individual can adjust to social standards and mix in. This is somebody who looks odd, in any believable way, while now and again offbeat, fiercely liberal or defiant. These people are regularly tall and etheric, or just anxious and restless more often than not. The best challenge of each Aquarius is to discover their center and the focal point of their character, loaded up with deference for their own needs and characters of everybody around them. They will neglect to see the motivation behind power and need to comprehend that sovereignty, just as sorting out and overseeing, are fundamental and helpful in their life. They are controlled by Saturn and Uranus.

The First House in Pisces

At the point when the primary house starts in the indication of Pisces, we need to comprehend this is an individual on a strategic, with a higher reason that should be perceived. This is somebody fine, touchy, passionate, with enormous eyes and a delicate soul. Frequently, this is an indication that gives a grieved physical make-up, particularly influencing one's psychological state. So as to utilize the best indication of Pisces brings to the table, an individual must have enough confidence, and a solid premise in childhood and training to satisfy their unbelievably enormous hunger for joy. Every one of these people needs to acknowledge desk work, sound idea, and reality in its most perfect and most evident structure. They need to figure out how to deal with subtleties and spotlight on explicit little things so as to make a greater picture with quality. Careful discipline brings about promising results, and this is something they ought to consistently recollect. Their rulers are Jupiter and Neptune.

Second House

On an individual level, this is the house that speaks to the worth we provide for ourselves and all that we do. In it, we can emerge our vitality into something we can contact, use, or grasp, as though it was a characteristic outcome of the vitality we help in our body spoke to through our first house. The second place of our graph is the field of propensity, the nourishment we eat, with the reason to bolster our yearning made by the creature we convey in the primary house. It is a wellspring of salary that fortifies our body, prompting considerations with quality. It associates with the indication of Taurus, talks about one's riches, and is additionally called the place of significant worth. Its Latin saying is Lucrum, signifying "riches."

The Second House in Aries

On the off chance that the subsequent house starts in the indication of Aries, we can see that this individual pursues their senses to make something in the material world. Aries on the second house cusp can talk about an individual's failure to appreciate things that are moderate, enjoyable, comfortable, or delicate. This can be a harsh position that structures an unpleasant character, except if ladylike planets and the Moon are emphatically situated in their horoscope.

The Second House in Taurus

The second house cusp in Taurus is the most common situation for this house. Individuals brought into the world with it can perceive the estimation of all things, connections, other individuals, and encounters throughout everyday life. At times, this talks about a complemented test wherein an individual should find out about their own an incentive through a progression of belittling encounters. In any case, this is once in a while the case. This must be affirmed through a difficult situation of Venus in one's natal graph. This is somebody who has the ability to acquire cash, for whatever length of time that their feeling of the material world isn't corrupted with other individuals' feelings and conclusions. In the event that they surrender to blame of any sort, the nature of their connections will abruptly drop and they could experience considerable difficulties recouping from assuming an excessive amount of liability. These people were destined to make the most of our material reality and ought to consistently remind themselves to do only that.

The Second House in Gemini

On the off chance that the subsequent house is set in the indication of Gemini, we can right away assume that an individual will profit in brisk, independent exercises, as opposed to have a genuine activity that will bring a great deal of profound, stable fulfillment. This is somebody who can benefit from composing, news coverage, steady development, rhetoric gifts, or great exchanging aptitudes. On the off chance that there is a test to be looked through planets set in this house or Mercury, we can see that shallow ways to deal with estimation of things lead to disharmony and make an individual apprehensive and tense, while unfit to make anything steady or enormous enough to address their issues. This can likewise speak to a "swindler position" and talk about somebody who profits from obscure exercises, particularly if Mercury is retrograde, or set in the indication of Pisces.

The Second House in Cancer

In the event that the subsequent house starts in the indication of Cancer, this is a solid sign that an individual will get an opportunity to acquire from a privately-run company or a privately owned business of their own. This is somebody skilled to telecommute, or somebody who takes the path of least resistance and depends on fate to present to them their riches. When all is said in done, this probably won't be such a solid position if the Moon isn't extremely solid, however enables to discover amazing happiness in nourishment, cooking, and family social events. This is a place that accents one's internal quest for appreciation and love, and it will regularly talk about hereditary inclinations as a potential for individual addition. It can likewise be a place that talks about legacy they have been going through since the day they were conceived, rather than legacy matters of the eighth house in which somebody needs amazing abandon something with the end goal for addition to come.

The Second House in Leo

In the event that an individual's second house cusp is set in the indication of Leo, we can see the capacity to posture for cash and this is regularly found in models, on-screen characters, and individuals who must be dramatic so as to get something for themselves. Contingent upon the poise of its ruler, this is the subsequent house position that talks about solid certainty with regards to material issues, however it can likewise make an individual powerless against other individuals' assessments with regards to their very own worth.

The Second House in Virgo

In the event that the subsequent house starts in the indication of Virgo, it is protected to assume this is somebody who has some things to find out about fulfillment. This is an indication that carries Venus to its fall, and since Venus is a characteristic ruler for maters of the subsequent house, we can see that the test here is to really esteem one's activities and victories, rather than scanning for deficiencies in all that they do. In the event that when solid Mercury hues this position, we can see somebody normal and proficient to fix whatever comes their direction. Be that as it may, it is as yet uncommon to discover an individual with this setting who is really happy with what they claim.

The Second House in Libra

At the point when the subsequent house is set in the indication of Libra, this gives an individual a feeling of self-esteem through associations with other individuals. As it were, this can be tricky and lead to envy and a wide range of evaluations that the Soul isn't prepared for, while simultaneously giving one a ton of material endowments through organizations or a picked mate. In an ineffectively set position, this can make an individual see their accomplice thought their assets, vain and went to the things of other individuals.

The Second House in Scorpio

On the off chance that the subsequent house has a cusp in the indication of Scorpio, this discusses funds left to us by our predecessors. Contingent upon our hereditary inclinations, this can be a gift or a revile, since it significantly relies upon those that were here before we resulted in these present circumstances world. It may appear as though we have little effect alone prosperity when this setting dominates. So as to discover bliss in the material world, this is a place that moves an individual to discover it in change and acknowledge that the vitality needs to stream and hover consistently. In the reasonable sense, this implies one needs to give so as to get and there will never come a reward without it being earned through a wide range of deeds, life decisions, and family. This is additionally a place that can talk about an obligation that must be reimbursed and it isn't in every case simple to grasp or appreciate.

The Second House in Sagittarius

On the off chance that the subsequent house discovered its cusp in the indication of Sagittarius, it is difficult to clutch cash or stick to beaten trails to gain it. Despite the fact that this is clearly somebody who can benefit from instructing, theory, or travel, the amount earned won't be effectively contained and will be spent rapidly. In spite of the fact that there is constantly a ton of karma where valuable Sagittarius is, there are numerous ridiculous methodologies and a propensity to exaggerate whatever the imagery of the house in question. This is actually why these individuals will in general eat excessively, spend excessively, just as gain excessively, or be in any capacity ridiculous about their own value and the estimation of the things they do and their achievements.

The Second House in Capricorn

On the off chance that one's horoscope conveys the second house cusp in the indication of Capricorn, this is regularly observed as a cross of fate that can't be changed. The best issue here lies in the blame conveyed somewhere down in one's spirit that prompts deplorable conditions and missteps made in the field of accounts or their dietary patterns. This isn't a place that will pardon a lot, particularly on the off chance that one isn't prepared to take on the majority of the duty regarding their life and their money related or material assets.

The Second House in Aquarius

In situations where the subsequent house starts in the indication of Aquarius, matters of significant worth will always show signs of change. The main consistent worth the individual will perceive will be found in their kinships and shared objectives of the general public, while it will be quite difficult to stay stable in one money related methodology. This is an individual that has a need to go for broke, much the same as they will go out on a limb with their wellbeing and every one of the things their body can deal with expending quick and lousy nourishment way over and over again for their liver and heart to take in. Much of the time, the primary place of somebody brought into the world with this subsequent house position is set in Capricorn, adding another measurement to the utilization of their vitality when making anything in the material world. Stable and with a solid arrangement, they appear to discover freedom through cash and this will frequently make them oddly flippant and brimming with shocks in every single monetary issue.

The Second House in Pisces

At the point when the subsequent house is situated in the indication of Pisces, numerous possessions will get lost now and again. This is found in somebody who doesn't have the foggiest idea where their keys are, much the same as they aren't sure where or when they will have the option to procure something all alone. The entangled thing here lies in the way that hallucinations with Pisces will in general dominate, and one can feel really and profoundly fulfilled without having a lot, much the same as they could overestimate their capacities in specific fields, lost in their actual strategic concentration towards material objectives.

Third House

The third house is additionally called "The House of Communications" and its adage means "siblings" from the Latin expression Fratres. It identifies with the indication of Gemini on an increasingly close to home, physical level, and talks about the inner parts of our brain. The primary concern its situating depicts is the way one thinks and the procedures in our minds that lead us a specific way. All things considered, it is critical in close to home graph investigation, for it gives us the data on an individual's perspective, much the same as the principal house discusses the condition of one's body, or the fourth the condition of feelings and heart.

The Third House in Aries

In the event that the third house begins in the indication of Aries, we see a person with a quick personality and a forceful way to deal with correspondence. This is somebody stimulated and loaded up with dynamic thoughts, whose psyche works constantly. It is a gift as much as it tends to be a revile, for the indication of Aries holds our uncertain annoyance gives the same amount of as it brings speed, insight, and clear thinking.

The Third House in Taurus

With the third house cusp in Taurus, musings are frequently moderate, static, and went to gluttonous or material issues. This is one of the most down to earth and useful positions, albeit once in a while aggravating for individuals with third house cusp in signs that have a place with the component of Air.

The Third House in Gemini

The situation of the third house in Gemini is the most normal everything being equal. It is a gift in itself, and an individual consistently has a savvy approach, clearness in their selection of words, and a similar lucidity in their psyche. In a commonsense sense, it regularly discusses one's connection to their kin and brings up that correspondence is a significant piece of an individual's life. Contingent upon the position and the pride of Mercury, we can perceive how testing or positive their psychological world really is.

The Third House in Cancer

The third house in Cancer talks about acquired insight, for better or in negative ways. In the event that one is naturally introduced to a group of accomplished people with a wide word reference, we can securely assume that theirs will be comparative and profoundly established in their heritage. Be that as it may, issues with any kind of thinking, particularly with regards to the division of sane from intense subject matters, have the root in a similar spot as well – their folks. They have to manufacture a solid character and care for their independence so as to discharge some weight from their brains.

The Third House in Leo

At the point when the third house cusp is set in the indication of Leo, musings are for the most part centered around one's Self. Despite the fact that this can be disturbing to numerous fellowships and dubious connections in their lives, these people have an errand to develop their character and character with unmistakably set limits towards the external world. This is a solid position that brings a ton of self-image difficulties, except if one is really edified and completely mindful of their limitless capacities, incorporating the one wherein they comprehend that there is nothing that ought to be taken actually.

The Third House in Virgo

On the off chance that the third house is set in Virgo, this is a peculiar position that is as frequently debilitating as much as it is engaging. While the indication of Virgo lifts up Mercury and talks about insight and fantastic mental capacities and clearness, it is additionally a point of commonsense issues, matters of physiology and schedule, and medical problems that don't should be examined.

The Third House in Libra

At the point when the third house is set in the indication of Libra, we can see somebody who thinks and talks about other people time and again. As much as this position can be beneficial for one's adoration life, talking about youth darlings, attractive neighbors, and the capacity to see "the opposite side of every story", it is additionally a test to go to their very own internal center except if they are appropriately worked through their childhood. This is somebody who must have a solid character, constantly mindful of their own judgment and frames of mind, before conversing with any other individual about them.

The Third House in Scorpio

At the point when the third house begins in Scorpio, it is rarely effectively taken care of. This is a solid, profound personality, regularly enhanced with a feeling of dim amusingness, and musings and words that are hard to stay unadulterated and free of disappointment. This position is a solid one for science, research, and mysterious issues, however, it gets difficulties regions of the heart and enthusiastic contacts with the nearest individuals. The haziness of Scorpio is best observed through one's psyche and an individual needs profound passionate lucidity and enough giggling and ease in life to acknowledge it with effortlessness and magnificence.

The Third House in Sagittarius

With the third house in Sagittarius, we in a split second observe somebody who rambles. This is a situation for philosophical masterminds and individuals of wide viewpoints, suppositions that consistently move to progressively positive perspectives, and the capacity to utilize their convictions to the extent of their useful presence. It can likewise discuss arrangements that consistently appear to be inaccessible, in the event that absence of course in life is highlighted and one has no learning of their own actual way and goal.

The Third House in Capricorn

With the third house beginning in Capricorn, we can see a truly extreme person. Despite the fact that Capricorn is the indication of profundity and levelheaded decisions just as the down to earth utilization of everything throughout everyday life, it is additionally an indication of karma, harmed things, and missteps of the heart. To keep your third house in Capricorn balance, you can't separate from your passionate center. Empathy pursued by rest is the way into any test of this house, particularly in situations where kin has consistent, interminable issues, regardless of on the off chance that they are material, physical, or some other kind.

The Third House in Aquarius

At the point when the third house has a place with the indication of Aquarius, we right away observe an amazing personality loaded up with splendid thoughts and a rich public activity. This is an agitator that never depends on the guidance of others and falls into the field of issues on the off chance that they start sustaining their conscience through perpetual counsel they will in general give. The significant thing to recognize here is that everybody is shrewd in their own particular manner, and no one needs any counsel given except if they explicitly requested it.

The Third House in Pisces

On the off chance that the third house is set in Pisces, we need to remember this is an indication of Mercury's fall. The best clash of feeling and reason is seen here, and it tends to confound, weird, and profoundly trying for one's capacity to talk, compose, or even think unmistakably.

Fourth House

The fourth house is the place of home and family. It is our most profound passionate center, our underlying foundations, and our hereditary legacy, as observed through the family tree and our predecessors with the majority of their relationship issues, clashes, fears, and dreams. It is a strange and our most typical, our place of propensity and association with the center of the Earth, similarly as it is our capacity to discover unbounded, genuine love, and consistent closeness to another person. This is the house that identifies with the indication of Cancer, and its Latin saying genitor means "parent", as though it was set for demonstrating the significance of one individual that made us feel comfortable, regardless of in the event that it is our genuine parent or essentially – ourselves.

The Fourth House in Aries

At the point when somebody has the fourth house cusp set in the indication of Aries, it regularly talks about the anxiety of a parent of the contrary sex when the graph's proprietor was as yet a child. If there should be an occurrence of an ideal situating, this is an indication of searing passionate clearness, speed of choices and the certainty one brought from their home and their childhood.

The Fourth House in Taurus

On the off chance that the fourth house is set in Taurus, we see a characteristic situation of consideration and physical dedication originating from one's folks. In spite of the fact that it can indicate out conventional or severe childhood, it generally furnishes one with a specific feeling of solace and satisfaction that makes a solid, fixed reason for a wonderful life.

The Fourth House in Gemini

With the fourth house cusp in Gemini, we can see the alterable and somewhat shaky nature of one's home. All the time, this comes as a root for an individual's inclination of irregularity, seen through conceivable contemptibility of their equivalent sex parent, or the picture of two dads or two moms, that they can't repair into one.

The Fourth House in Cancer

Every fourth house set in Cancer discusses the association one has to their family. It is a place of legacy in its center, and the indication of Cancer here gives an accentuation on family matters that came into one's life just to be settled.

The Fourth House in Leo

With the fourth house starting in the indication of Leo, we see a line of glad and daring precursors that prompted the introduction of this person. This can be superb or trying for there is clearly an enthusiastic push into one's universe of character, certainty, and self-acknowledgment.

The Fourth House in Virgo

The fourth house cusp in Virgo indicates the absence of something in their essential home. Regardless of whether it is love or endorsement, there consistently is by all accounts something that should be fixed, changed, or sustained in their spirit, as though it was somewhat harmed from the beginning.

The Fourth House in Libra

On the off chance that the fourth is set in Libra, we see somebody who conveys a solid premise of their folks' relationship in their most profound center. Since the fourth house speaks to our home, we immediately comprehend this is an individual whose house was adjusted and apparently upbeat, yet the fundamental issue of Libra is the irregularity of the picture that appeared to the outside world and the genuine delight holed up behind it.

The Fourth House in Scorpio

With the fourth house in Scorpio, we can see the most grounded connections to a family that regularly aren't sound or sincerely steady. Scorpio is an indication that carries the Moon to its fall, and all things considered isn't in the best relationship to issues of family, child-rearing, childhood, and closeness.

The Fourth House in Sagittarius

With the fourth house in Sagittarius, it isn't actually simple to feel comfortable, any place one attempts to settle. This is one of the difficulties prompting life abroad, regularly in light of the fact that there were separation and space in their childhood that makes it difficult to consolidate their convictions into the nation they were conceived in.

The Fourth House in Capricorn

There is no motivation to make it prettier than it is – the fourth house in Capricorn is rarely simple. In the most ideal situation, this is a place that gives one definitive confidence in the Universe, and a solid association with God. With a profoundly seeded need to assume liability, this is a person who frequently takes a lot of it, for the most part snatching some for each mix-up made by their folks.

The Fourth House in Aquarius

With the fourth house in Aquarius, an individual consistently is by all accounts looking for consistency. This is a sign there was a great deal of moving and changes at a youthful age or calls attention to the significance of the separation guardians experienced while they were still in the period of enthusiastic acknowledgment with their youngster.

The Fourth House in Pisces

It is regularly said that the fourth house in Pisces discusses the record pieces of information and obscure progenitors that have done who-recognizes what. Be that as it may, this can in some cases just talk about the absence of lucidity of feeling one gets in their essential condition.

Fifth House

Individual articulation stows away in this house and anything in great connection to it will enable one to develop, develop, and discover genuine fulfillment in this lifetime through exercises that will fill their vitality pool and make them feel invigorated. All shades of the world are set in this house, and this is actually why we have to locate its best imagery and the most grounded indicate all together arrive at genuine innovativeness and express through something helpful and excellent. Its Latin aphorism Nati means "youth", alluding not exclusively to the kids we raise yet to our own kid inside.

The Fifth House in Aries

It is continually strengthening and fulfilling to have the fifth house set in a Fire sign. Moreover, Aries is an indication that lifts up the Sun and in association with this house. It talks about one's solid life power, certainty, and activity in a quest for satisfaction.

The Fifth House in Taurus

With the fifth house in the indication of Taurus, it is entirely expected to assume that one's fulfillment lies in money related and material things. In any case, it is fairly an account of Venus and we can't state that it principally discusses cash. This is somebody who needs to discover euphoria in the material world, and such a position will regularly talk about the affection for nourishment and indulging as a way to cover disappointments that absence of activity keeps them from settling.

The Fifth House in Gemini

On account of the fifth house set in Gemini, we can see somebody whose kid inside is genuinely adolescent and garrulous. It is very simple to identify with kids with this position, and become mindful of one's actual motivations, thought processes, and character at a youthful age.

The Fifth House in Cancer

At the point when one's fifth house is set in the indication of Cancer, fulfillment is constantly discovered someplace in the family tree. This can be as satisfying as it very well may challenge, for one's close to home articulation and delight appear to depend incredibly on their precursors and their degree of awareness.

The Fifth House in Leo

The fifth house in the indication of Leo speaks to a characteristic guideline that unequivocally stresses one's character. The manly, beneficial vitality of Leo must be utilized, and the most noticeably terrible thing these people can do is attempt to adjust to the assessments of individuals around them and end up in an exacting daily schedule with no space for their red hot articulation.

The Fifth House in Virgo

With the fifth house in Virgo, the principal challenge is to maintain a strategic distance from self-analysis on an approach to satisfaction. Happiness is found in subtleties, in things well-done, and everything that necessities fixing and extra consideration. This is the fifth place of commonsense issues and it is somewhat difficult to fulfill, yet very compensating with regards to composing and articulation through explicit words and manual work.

The Fifth House in Libra

At the point when the fifth house is set in the indication of Libra, we see a solid sign that satisfaction is come to through other individuals. This is to some degree trying for autonomy should be supported all together for any character to arrive at solid advancement, however, it is additionally important to show oneself through other individuals and focus on everybody that fulfills one en route.

The Fifth House in Scorpio

The fifth house set in the indication of Scorpio discusses the affection for profound passionate difficulties. To comprehend somebody who conveys this situation in their natal outline, we need to comprehend the need for progress, torment, enslavement, dread, and at last demise.

The Fifth House in Sagittarius

At the point when the fifth house is set in Sagittarius, we see that an individual has an incredible love for theory, travel, instructing, and training. As a rule, this is a decent sign that will enable one to create and remain open for wide lessons and a wide range of points of view changed on their way to satisfaction.

The Fifth House in Capricorn

At the point when the fifth house is in the indication of Capricorn, the challenges of dread, frenzy, fit, and a conspicuous absence of rest that appear to live here. It is never simple to have the fifth house here, as it empties a ton of vitality out of an individual and talks about the failure to appreciate, have some good times, and offer joyful and light exercises with other individuals.

The Fifth House in Aquarius

Aquarius is an indication of advancements, higher correspondences, and the system we are largely unknowingly wired to, so this is frequently a sign that somebody has a solid drive to make something unprecedented, unique, new, and unfathomable on the off chance that they just figure out how to express their actual inward character.

The Fifth House in Pisces

With the fifth house starting in Pisces, an individual certainly has an ability that should be found and utilized. Whatever they discover a love for will turn into their wellspring of motivation, and despite the fact that the indication of Pisces is variable and not entirely steady all things considered, this is constantly a pointer to incredible love, one we've met in our previous existences.

Sixth House

The Sixth place of every horoscope speaks to the transporter of wellbeing and physiological issues and conditions in this lifetime. It is the condition of our body with its vitality and stamina characterized by the principal house. Whatever the circumstance displayed through our 6th house, our assumptions need to discover affirmation through the power of issues or characteristics of the Ascendant and its ruler, for they give out the primary physical picture and our base, carnal qualities and shortcomings. In its center, the 6th place of a natal graph is a position of schedule that gives us great sustenance, wellbeing, and fulfillment, relating to the indication of Virgo and talking about our viable, regular daily existence. Its Latin maxim is Valetudo, signifying "wellbeing", characterizing this as its essential job in our diagram.

The Sixth House in Aries

At the point when the 6th house begins in the indication of Aries, we see somebody whose vitality is firmly connected to their working daily practice. This is a place that puts an emphasis on one's have to rehearse, start something new, practice day by day, and for the most part, talks about the vitality rise that is activated by changes to one's daily schedule.

The Sixth House in Taurus

With the 6th house starting in Taurus, we see a basic test of nourishment, which means it is basic to locate a decent daily practice in this lifetime, eat well while additionally making the most of what's on the table in the most ideal manner.

The Sixth House in Gemini

The 6th house in Gemini talks about one's psychological inhabitance and the capacity, or the powerlessness, to isolate from the universe of a creative mind and thought, and come down to this present reality where establishing is found.

The Sixth House in Cancer

The 6th house in Cancer interfaces one's profound passionate roots to the place of work and wellbeing. It likewise talks about the oblivious propensities that lead to specific conditions and down to earth conditions.

The Sixth House in Leo

With the 6th house set in Leo, silly bliss should be found in the work environment. This is a place that stresses physical quality somehow or another, and its indication is, for the most part, observed through the situation of the Sun.

The Sixth House in Virgo

The 6th house sees its regular situation like the one in Virgo. The association between them is amazingly solid and establishing found through this connection is genuinely basic in one's life.

The Sixth House in Libra

With the 6th house in Libra, the way into one's wellbeing lies to be determined, as in everything associated with Libra. With enough data these people get the chance to eat healthy, assuming liability for their state and effectively adjusting to new workplaces.

The Sixth House in Scorpio

On the off chance that the 6th house is set in the indication of Scorpio, pointless conduct is the best foe to one's physiology and mental state. Difficulties that stow away in this position are not in the least simple to deal with, for their center rests in passionate disappointment, absolution, and change. On the off chance that there is forswearing, expulsion, and obstruction towards change, Scorpio won't make one upbeat and a great deal of outrage will collect here.

The Sixth House in Sagittarius

The 6th house in Sagittarius is in its premise a defensive power for somebody's wellbeing. This is a position held by individuals with enormous pets, huge objectives, and dreams that can be brought practical by a basic arrangement of feelings. The whole association of life, for the most part, relies upon an individual's concentration and the capacity to locate the correct calling and the correct bearing.

The Sixth House in Capricorn

With the 6th house in Capricorn, rest and a dull routine are the main things that can enable one to recapture the vitality and feel sure and solid. A profession is by all accounts reliant on external conditions, specialists that are difficult to acknowledge, and this is incredibly testing if the Sun has any kind of issue with Uranus, Aquarius, or the eleventh house ruler.

The Sixth House in Aquarius

At the point when the indication of Aquarius is at the 6th house cusp, it is constantly a sign that a normal found in the essential family isn't solid or supporting for the physiology of the individual. Changes are vital and cheap food, light rest, and mental distraction won't support the pressure or issues with nerves.

The Sixth House in Pisces

With the 6th house in Pisces, there is something obscure about the way to deal with a sound way of life. Vitality can get truly low and reality can begin appearing to be blurred and lost as though it was difficult to keep the two feet on the ground anyway hard one may attempt.

Seventh House

Matters of the seventh house are constantly set in the outside world and connections we will in general make. Its Latin saying is Uxor and this means "life partner" with its particular job as a mirror to our own Self found in other individuals. This relates to the indication of Libra speaking to our basic parity and our capacity to interface with others in the nearest conceivable manner. This manifestation gives us the assignment to discover harmony in connection to something explicit, and this is seen through the sign on the seventh house cusp, planets inside this house, and its ruler.

The Seventh House in Aries

With the seventh house set in the indication of Aries, affability isn't seen frequently in cozy connections. There is continually something covered up in the way of life of contention that should be educated, and the most commonplace situation talks about one's propensity to reject the advantages of contention, keeping away from it despite the fact that it would be useful and helpful.

The Seventh House in Taurus

With the seventh house in Taurus, there is constantly a test of different sides of Venus in the field of connections. Taurus is an indication of pragmatic qualities and grounded, natural magnificence, some of the time unreasonably basic for "pedigreed" people went to fine, touchy, external excellence. The seventh house is comparing to the indication of Libra, and in that capacity discusses external magnificence, cosmetics, posture, and vanity in its difficulties.

The Seventh House in Gemini

On the off chance that the seventh house is set in Gemini, there is clearly a great deal to discuss in this lifetime. This is an individual who considers correspondence to be key to any circumstance nearby. Closeness is come to through discussions, individuals are met at parties, and the picture of a loquacious companion is regularly excessively highlighted.

The Seventh House in Cancer

On the off chance that the seventh house starts in the indication of Cancer, there is a great deal left in the field of connections from our precursors and family. It is practically difficult to isolate one's close to home objectives and bonds framed with other individuals from those of guardians and close relatives that introduced good examples in the individual's childhood.

The Seventh House in Leo

With the seventh house in Leo, all connections depend exclusively on an individual's capacity to locate a center ground and a point of concurrence with others as opposed to trading off pointlessly and going to limits of doing and not doing what others need.

The Seventh House in Virgo

The seventh house set in the indication of Virgo talks about quietude and carries center to issues of analysis, the capacity to discover fulfillment in reality and structure connections that don't need to be impeccable so as to last.

The Seventh House in Libra

This is a characteristic situation of the seventh house, prompting a characteristic way to deal with connections, marriage and a capacity to be careful and political towards others, regardless of on the off chance that they are our companions or foes.

The Seventh House in Scorpio

With the seventh house set in the indication of Scorpio, extreme closeness is required all together for the individual to discover fulfillment. This is a position extremely difficult to please and the idea of the principal house as of now demonstrates the capacity to make delicate closeness and closeness, normally rejected and decreased by others.

The Seventh House in Sagittarius

On the off chance that the seventh house is set in Sagittarius, its impermanent idea meddles with one's capacity to shape enduring connections.

The Seventh House in Capricorn

Despite the fact that the seventh house in Capricorn regularly talks about limitations and characters that are difficult to consolidate with one's center character, it gives a specific awareness of other's expectations and tolerance towards other individuals.

The Seventh House in Aquarius

Aquarius is an indication that discusses separation and division, just as all resistances that are consolidated in ideal agreement in nature around us.

The Seventh House in Pisces

At the point when the seventh house starts in Pisces, matters of trust are of most extreme significance for any solid connections an individual may have. Convictions will make fate, while there is frequently a type of mission one needs to satisfy so as to discover fulfillment and satisfaction.

Eight House

This is a house that conceals everything that is messy, our waste and our displeasure, our feelings, connections and things that we have to liberate from, just as all that we push under the carpet, declining to bargain. In its last sign, this is the place of death, coming as the stopping point after such a large number of things have been expelled for our body to deal with, yet additionally as an inescapable piece of life. It is additionally called the House of Reincarnation, while its Latin maxim Mors actually signifies "demise."

The Eighth House in Aries

With the eighth house in Aries, the principal challenge of life is to acknowledge the helpful power of annoyance and struggle. In the event that Mars isn't amazingly all around situated, this talks about one's propensity to squander their vitality on unimportant issues, these seen fundamentally through testing parts of Mars.

The Eighth House in Taurus

Taurus is an indication that commends life while the eighth house is the one to annihilate it. Perhaps the best restriction of the zodiac is found in this position and change will come as this moderate, troublesome obstruction with life that basically needs to break sooner or later.

The Eighth House in Gemini

With the eighth house in Gemini, changes consistently travel through one's psychological plain and shallow methodology is practically difficult to acknowledge. This is a run of the mill position for those brought into the world with their ascendant in Scorpio, and we will see that they experience genuine difficulty tolerating anything joyful that needs profundity and profound impulse in its center.

The Eighth House in Cancer

With the eighth house in Cancer, it is practically difficult to control internal apprehensions left as a legacy by our older folks. This is a run of the mill position for those whose moms feared pregnancy, might feel lost and desolate in their perspective.

The Eighth House in Leo

In the event that the eighth house is in Leo, there is no simple method to acknowledge authority. Not exclusively will an individual need a difference in close to home picture and view, yet they will likewise observe all sense of self-related issues of their own, in other individuals. In the event that they won't acknowledge the immature conduct and endeavors of others, this just means they are not destined for success.

The Eighth House in Virgo

The indication of Virgo has some thought about what indulgence is. It may also appear to want to go into a nitty-gritty examination of everything, removing from hues out of inventive things throughout everyday life. The primary issue is covered up in the way that without detail, there wouldn't be usefulness, and to ground any affected thought, we must be pragmatic enough to resolve to subtleties.

The Eighth House in Libra

The eighth house in Libra is a really weird situation for this is by all accounts connected to individuals who need to be separated from everyone else. Despite the fact that it is our regular need to have somebody to adore, going after immaculate congruity, this clearly doesn't make a difference to everybody in the zodiac.

The Eighth House in Scorpio

This is a place that effectively gathers all rubbish into one spot. There is a profoundly seeded information of endings and beginnings of everything throughout everyday life, while these people acknowledge the entire cycle of life and demise unique in relation to some other individuals in their lives.

The Eighth House in Sagittarius

At the point when the eighth house is set in Sagittarius, there is something peculiar about the feelings this individual has. Everything that they envision will work – won't, and the other way around, as though the whole Universe is there to show them the relativity of all things.

The Eighth House in Capricorn

On the off chance that the eighth house is set in Capricorn, duty is something that doesn't appear to have an incentive to the person. This can prompt a wide range of troublesome conditions in the event that Saturn is tested and there isn't sufficient rest and quiet encounters throughout their life.

The Eighth House in Aquarius

We are for the most part mindful of positive sides to the indication of Aquarius, particularly those of us who love Astrology or submit out a presence to it. Individuals with their eighth house set in Aquarius will, in general, observe just negative sides to this sign, and can't deal with the pressure, changes, the development of human advancement, and quick discussions that don't appear to have their establishing.

The Eighth House in Pisces

This can mean either that they are excessively levelheaded in their regular conditions to offer an incentive to their fantasies, or that every one of their endeavors to appear their wants fall flat.

Ninth House

The ninth house is the place of theory, point of view, and travel. Its Latin adage Iter means "adventures" and this is actually what this house talks about. It is a position of higher personality and comprehension past everything found in our material world, past our limits and points of confinement of our body.

The Ninth House in Aries

At the point when the ninth house is in the indication of Aries, an individual can be too enthusiastic about their convictions, not enabling others to express their arrangement of feelings. Warriors for religion, moral methodology, school, or their very own advancement of any sort are seen here.

The Ninth House in Taurus

In the event that the ninth house is set in Taurus, the motivation behind an individual's life is constantly discovered someplace in the material world. Experience should be worked in reality, through monetary and physical issues, and this is the accurate motivation behind why these people go to training in fields of money, farming, cooking, or land.

The Ninth House in Gemini

The ninth house in Gemini prompts development through correspondence. These people will adapt to new things rapidly and with enthusiasm, while simultaneously experiencing difficulty clutching enormous pieces of information or discovering amalgamation for all that they've learned. To patch the issues found in overthinking, they have to likewise figure out how to remain compact and concentrated on each point in turn.

The Ninth House in Cancer

With the ninth house in Cancer, there is constantly a straightforward endeavoring held in an individual's way – to discover harmony. This isn't a simple strategic somebody with their mind holding up traffic, for our human instinct frequently doesn't enable enough quietness and harmony to arrive at that truly necessary condition of lucidity and harmony.

The Ninth House in Leo

At the point when the ninth house is set in the indication of Leo, we see that somebody needs to explain the picture of self separated from their family, childhood, and qualities educated at home. On the off chance that they are too pleased to even think about accepting that fact is comparative with all individuals, they can end up pushy and power their conclusions and feelings on everybody around them.

The Ninth House in Virgo

The ninth house in Virgo discusses the emphasis on helping other people, philanthropy work, and matters of humility and detail. The individuals who were brought into the world with this house position regularly want to figure out how to recuperate and normally comprehend the knowledge of their physiology and pragmatic issues in the material world.

The Ninth House in Libra

On the off chance that the ninth house is set in Libra, there is something abnormally confounding in an individual's conviction framework, the fundamental issue is the way that their convictions appear to be characterized by other individuals. They will discover numerous good examples in this lifetime and need to beat their self-analysis so as to really arrive at their ideal perspective, physical state, or expert objectives that they see as their calling.

The Ninth House in Scorpio

With the ninth house in Scorpio, we need to comprehend that an individual will settle on decisions that many would consider as odd. In the best sign, this will give one an unimaginable profundity of the brain, confidence in the intensity of planet Earth, association with unlimited pools of inward vitality and a propensity to think about science, brain science, or even mysterious lessons.

The Ninth House in Sagittarius

The ninth house in the indication of Sagittarius talks about a higher personality, as it were, and demonstrates one's have to travel, learn, and enlarge their points of view however much as could reasonably be expected.

The Ninth House in Capricorn

On the off chance that one's ninth house is set in the indication of Capricorn, their convictions can be annoyingly hardened. It will be difficult for them to roll out an improvement in pace or heading once they set out to accomplish something. Their fundamental issue is covered up in a genuine reason for everything in their lives. This is the reason they now and again need to trade their reasonableness and sound judgment for a fantasy or two.

The Ninth House in Aquarius

With the ninth house in Aquarius, one's strivings and wants are rarely standard. Learning through images will be at least somewhat simple, makes these individuals went to crystal gazing, science, and programming. The issue will emerge when an individual with this ninth house doesn't want to acknowledge obligation regarding their very own life.

The Ninth House in Pisces

On the off chance that somebody's ninth house is set in the indication of Pisces, there is unquestionably a strategic ought to follow in this lifetime.

Tenth House

At the point when we talk about our vocation and our economic wellbeing, we are talking about our tenth house. It is where the majority of our aspirations go, and simply like Mars is magnified in the tenth sign – Capricorn, our first house ruler normally centers around our tenth house to arrive at its objectives. Its Latin witticism regnum signifies "Kingdom" and serves well for us to comprehend the significance of this house in our own life.

The Tenth House in Aries

On the off chance that the tenth house is set in the indication of Aries, there is a characteristic required for an individual to concentrate their vitality on vocation objectives and the material future they can assemble. This is the position associated with trailblazers and the individuals who began something new, ending up generally known due to their drive and their capacity to lead the way.

The Tenth House in Taurus

With the tenth house in Taurus, an individual's objective in life is by all accounts physical, arousing fulfillment. The situation of Venus will let us know of the everyday issue this applies to, yet it will consistently be associated with the quest for sexual joy and the right, sound daily practice.

The Tenth House in Gemini

If the tenth house is set in Gemini, we can immediately assume that an individual likes to talk and be seen talking. Similarly, as the seventh house, Gemini likes to impart their insights with the world, this is somebody who offers as well as gives data a chance to characterize them in the public eye.

The Tenth House in Cancer

At the point when the tenth house is in Cancer, we see that jobs have been turned around, and the family this individual needs to make looks like enormously of the family they originated from. Enthusiastic and expert are interwoven here, so it is very ordinary for them to keep maintaining a privately-owned company, or turn their lives towards youngsters and the picture of an ideal family.

The Tenth House in Leo

With the tenth house in Leo, you get an ordinary chief. Regardless of whether this individual isn't gifted to administer individuals and their Sun is powerless, they will even now attempt to flaunt and present themselves as prevailing, solid, huge, or as though they are the ones who rule.

The Tenth House in Virgo

At the point when the tenth house is in the indication of Virgo, an individual is by all accounts brought into the world with a need to fix their objectives. They will infrequently reach skyward enough or pursue positions they may have been made as though they go to self-judgment too simple to even think about making any expert advancement whatsoever.

The Tenth House in Libra

If the tenth house is set in Libra, we in a flash observe that the focal point of one's reality is found in their connections. Other individuals will characterize the goal this individual will pick, and it won't be simple on their character if the Sun isn't solid in its position and manner through the planet administering it.

The Tenth House in Scorpio

If somebody's tenth house starts in the indication of Scorpio, the primary concern they should reach in this lifetime is enthusiastic profundity. This is a profound Water sign that permits no shallow emotions, and in that capacity, it is a solid reason for expert achievement.

The Tenth House in Sagittarius

With the tenth house in Sagittarius, it is obvious that learning prompts progress as though life was a basic condition. Be that as it may, this is the indication all things considered and it demonstrates the propensity of an individual to work abroad or pursue their profession objectives someplace a long way from the spot they were conceived in.

The Tenth House in Capricorn

At the point when the tenth house starts in Capricorn desire isn't an issue and things will, in general, be as quite obvious. The issue will emerge once the individual understands that their absence of vitality prompted some terrible decisions, pushing them into pointless sentiments of blame.

The Tenth House in Aquarius

On the off chance that the tenth house is in Aquarius, an individual is quite often capricious, extraordinary, wearing hues you don't see each day, or in another route abnormal to the external world.

The Tenth House in Pisces

At the point when the tenth house is in Pisces, there is no truism to what extent their profession decisions will last. This is frequently baffling as the reason for each activity gradually blurs accounting for commitments and obligations an individual isn't prepared to sink into.

Eleventh House

This is a place of kinship yet, in addition, this weird point in a horoscope where we discover approaches to speak with our inward character and the external Universe. The eleventh house essentially speaks to how God addresses us. This is our view of confidence, convictions, religion, and everything that offers a reason to our reality. It will push us towards accommodating exercises and decisions made for the prosperity of the whole humankind. Its Latin name Benefacta means "fellowship" and this is, unquestionably, its essential job.

The Eleventh House in Aries

At the point when the eleventh house starts in Aries, things are never tranquil in this present individual's public activity. There are in every case new associates holding up not far off, and this can make their methodology somewhat shallow given the conviction life will continually bring another person our way. It will be anything but difficult to make companions yet somewhat difficult to clutch them for exceptionally long.

The Eleventh House in Taurus

The eleventh house in Taurus talks about the significance of public activity for an individual's material fulfillment. This doesn't mean their associations with companions have anything to do with cash, although they effectively could, yet rather than the fulfillments of the Earth are perceived through them. They will find out about their faculties through social contacts and frequently have many steady, cherishing and delicate connections that endure forever.

The Eleventh House in Gemini

With the eleventh house in Gemini, we see somebody who wishes to discuss has something to express and consistently finds a few people to tune in. Fellowships are quick, energizing and gutsy. There is constantly a ton to talk about and consider while conceptualizing is the most fulfilling movement in their social experiences.

The Eleventh House in Cancer

If the eleventh house starts in Cancer, everybody in this current individual's family will feel like companions. This is an odd situation, as the eleventh house ought to be there to liberate us from our enthusiastic ties, however, this isn't the situation here. These people have solid affections for those they associate with, have increased faculties around other individuals and treat others with compassion.

The Eleventh House in Leo

With the eleventh house in Leo, the picture of kinships effectively turns out to be a higher priority than genuine companions. On one hand, this is a significant issue in an individual's life, and on the other, they will, in general, mingle just with individuals who make them look great. Self-acknowledgment comes through other individuals and it tends to be hard to avoid control and individuals who force their will and show affront.

The Eleventh House in Virgo

At the point when the eleventh house is set in the indication of Virgo, there is regularly some kind of problem with companions this individual finds.

The Eleventh House in Libra

The eleventh house likes to be in Libra for its correspondence issues and its emphasis on significant connections making it simple to shape social contacts. Be that as it may, the indication of Libra itself doesn't appreciate this position prompting such a large number of changes in their passionate life, just as breakups or separation on the off chance that they haven't picked an accomplice who is both their companion and their darling consolidated.

The Eleventh House in Scorpio

While many would believe that the eleventh house in Scorpio is very troublesome and holding, we shouldn't overlook that the indication of Scorpio is the indication of the worship of Uranus and talks about the closest companions we could discover.

The Eleventh House in Sagittarius

On the off chance that the eleventh house is in the indication of Sagittarius, individuals who encompass this individual are promoters, educators, voyagers, and liberal companions who wouldn't fret contrasts in assessments, training or race.

The Eleventh House in Capricorn

At the point when the eleventh house starts in Capricorn, companionships last, loaded up with tolerance and a feeling of commitment. Without a solid premise, there is little that should be possible to improve public activity, and they should be encompassed by the individuals who come exceptionally "suggested" by those they as of now trust.

The Eleventh House in Aquarius

The eleventh house in Aquarius talks about freedom an individual needs. Captives to our unfortunate schedules, decisions, propensities, and connections, these individuals will have an unmistakable wish to be free and communicated as precisely themselves in their general public.

The Eleventh House in Pisces

At the point when the eleventh house is in the indication of Pisces, companionships are cloudy and misty. This is an individual who has an undertaking to discover confidence in others and it will consistently accompany difficulties and challenges in their manner.

Twelfth House

This is a house with the Latin name Carcer, signifying "jail" and it can truly transform your life into jail in any conceivable manner. It is additionally called The House of Self-Undoing. The regular advancement of our Self experiences that consistent column of houses, the second after the main, the third after the second, and so forth.

The Twelfth House in Aries

At the point when the twelfth house is set in the indication of Aries, it is quite often a sign that issues with sound limits will be available in an individual's life. Others will barge in their reality as though they had no layers to perceive and safeguard themselves from the individuals who take their vitality.

The Twelfth House in Taurus

On the off chance that the twelfth house is in the indication of Taurus, the secret of the material world can stay covered up for quite a long time, just as indulgence and the pursuit for fulfillment in this material world. This is a position ordinary for the individuals who have never felt genuine joy, and everybody with mystery sexual experiences, or if nothing else the individuals who want to eat escaped every other person.

The Twelfth House in Gemini

The twelfth house in Gemini isn't exceptionally simple in light of its Piscean nature and all that it has to do with feeling as an element completely separated from a sane idea. Discourse can be debilitated, while those with lower confidence effectively go to talk and matters that aren't theirs to examine in the first place. This is additionally a place that could give an awesome ability for dialects, words, and composing.

The Twelfth House in Cancer

With the twelfth house in the indication of Cancer, you can see an off the record piece of information in a split second, just as the inclination to admire either of the guardians. This is a weight of a whole family tree and an imprint that obligations were left in circles of the passionate and the delicate inside. Weird issues are stowing away in the twelfth house and when Cancer is here, you can see these bizarre issues in one's home and close connections.

The Twelfth House in Leo

At the point when the twelfth house starts in Leo, the character itself is by all accounts abnormal, delicate, and obscure. These people should find out about their capacity and their internal truth, while they stay in the hazy waters escaped plain sight.

The Twelfth House in Virgo

If the twelfth house is in Virgo, we can nearly envision the system in an individual's mind causing them to appear to be inept when they need to indicate how shrewd they are, and unimaginably savvy in the most eccentric circumstances.

The Twelfth House in Libra

With the twelfth house in Libra, it appears to be inescapable to lie or be misled, and normally both. In any case, on the off chance that we set this aside, we can see the supernatural story of Libra in this puzzling house and understand that somebody we once left behind is there for us to discover them again in this life. Things that were lost in our twelfth house tend to show themselves sometime in the not so distant future.

The Twelfth House in Scorpio

The twelfth house in Scorpio is an intriguing spot. Something as unthinkable and as covered up as Scorpio once in a while find a suitable undercover den, yet this position enables them to. The most disastrous thing here lies in one's capacity to cover their very own emotions, doings, or yearnings, at long last winding up with no attention to their actual inward light.

The Twelfth House in Sagittarius

At the point when the twelfth house is set in Sagittarius, we generally observe somebody who has no clue where they are going. Being lost is by all accounts the inborn ailment in these individuals and they have no chance to get of knowing where they need to wind up.

The Twelfth House in Capricorn

With the twelfth house in Capricorn, there is no knowing which duty falls under whose locale. The trouble of this setting covers up in the failure to see that a solid establishment makes all the work, and keeping in mind that smart thoughts can make some amazing progress, they aren't effectively appeared if diligent work isn't placed in.

The Twelfth House in Aquarius

The twelfth house in Aquarius talks about an unpleasant demise that occurred in our previous existence. This is a position of pressure and bizarre mental direction, pulling emphatically with its others conscious gravity and the oblivious need to liberate, set apart from every other person, and sink into every single common resistance as though there was no other way.

The Twelfth House in Pisces

On the off chance that the twelfth house is set in the indication of Pisces, all privileged insights will be sunk much more profound than in different cases. This implies all burrowing through intuitive issues should be intensive and results will appear to be more removed than those others will in general uncover.

Chapter 2

Getting To Know The 12 Zodiac Signs

Aries

As the main sign in the zodiac, the nearness of Aries consistently denotes the start of something vivacious and violent. They are persistently searching for dynamic, speed and rivalry, continually being the first in all things - from work to get-togethers. On account of its decision planet Mars and the reality it has a place with the component of Fire (simply like Leo and Sagittarius), Aries is one of the most dynamic zodiac signs. It is in their inclination to make a move, now and then before they consider it well.

The Sun in such high respect gives them great hierarchical abilities, so you'll once in a while meet an Aries who isn't equipped for completing a few things without a moment's delay, regularly before mid-day break! Their difficulties show when they get restless, forceful and vent outrage directing it toward other individuals. Solid characters brought into the world under this sign have an assignment to battle for their objectives, grasping fellowship and collaboration through this manifestation.

Aries governs the head and leads with the head, frequently actually strolling head first, inclining advances for speed and core interest. Its agents are normally daring and infrequently terrified of preliminary and hazard. They have energetic quality and vitality, paying little respect to their age and rapidly plays out some random errands.

The narrative of the Golden Fleece guides the Flying Ram. An Aries is prepared to be the saint of the day, fly away, and convey many jeopardized, frail individuals on their back. The intensity of the slam is carried on his back, for he is simply the gold, sparkly and appealing to those prepared for double-crossing. The tale of greatness that isn't anything but difficult to convey is in these two horns, and if this creature doesn't get shorn, permitting change and giving somebody a warm sweater, they won't have a lot to get from the world. Every Aries has an assignment to share their position, power, gold, or physical quality with other individuals enthusiastically, or the vitality will be halted in its characteristic stream, dread will dominate, and the way toward giving and accepting will hold the parity at zero.

Taurus

With common sense and a well-grounded attitude, Taurus is the sign that gathers the products of work. They want to consistently be encompassed by adoration and excellence. Individuals brought into the world with their Sun in Taurus are erotic and material, considering contact and taste the most significant everything being equal. Steady and preservationist, this is one of the most solid indications of the zodiac, prepared to suffer and adhere to their decisions until they arrive at the purpose of individual fulfillment.

Taurus is an Earth sign, much the same as Virgo and Capricorn, and can see things from a grounded, useful and sensible point of view. They think that its simple to profit and remain on similar ventures for a considerable length of time, or until they are finished. What we regularly observe as tenacity can be deciphered as responsibility, and their capacity to finish errands whatever it takes is uncanny. This makes them magnificent workers, incredible long haul companions and accomplices, continually being there for individuals they cherish. The natural note makes them overprotective, traditionalist, or materialistic now and again, with perspectives on the world established on their adoration for cash and riches.

56

The leading planet of Taurus is Venus, the planet of affection, fascination, magnificence, fulfillment, imagination, and appreciation. This delicate nature will make Taurus a phenomenal cook, nursery worker, sweetheart, and craftsman. They are steadfast and don't care for unexpected changes, analysis or the pursuit of blame individuals are regularly inclined to, being to some degree reliable on other individuals and feelings they appear to be not able relinquished. All things considered, regardless of their potential passionate test, these people can get a pragmatic voice of explanation of any turbulent and undesirable circumstances.

The Wandering Bull, being the person who sold out their closest companion, the goddess Hera herself, is a disastrous being that needs to meander the Earth to discover opportunity. As though something was continually jabbing them despite their good faith, helping them to remember the joy that used to be, stinging and pushing advances, they close up in their very own universes, forlorn and isolated from their center. To discover love, a Taurus needs to venture to the far corners of the planet, change the point of view or make a move in their whole conviction framework and their arrangement of qualities.

Gemini

Expressive and intelligent, Gemini speaks to two distinct characters in one and you will never be certain which one you will confront. They are friendly, informative and prepared for the sake of entertainment, with an inclination to abruptly quit fooling around, astute and anxious. They are captivated with the world itself, amazingly inquisitive, with a steady feeling that there isn't sufficient opportunity to encounter all that they need to see.

The indication of Gemini has a place with the component of Air, going with Libra and Aquarius, and this associates it to all parts of the brain.

It is governed by Mercury, the planet that speaks to correspondence, composing, and development. Individuals brought into the world under this Sun sign regularly have an inclination that their other half is missing, so they are always looking for new companions, coaches, partners, and individuals to converse with.

Gemini's alterable and receptive outlook makes them fantastic craftsmen, particularly authors and writers, and their abilities and adaptability make them sparkle in exchange, driving, and group activities. This is an adaptable, curious, carefree sign, brought into the world with a desire to encounter everything there is out there, on the planet. This makes their character motivating, and never exhausting.

There is so a lot of whimsical guiltlessness in the idea of Gemini, telling their story of fraternity, love between closest companions and relatives who are altogether unique by character, conditions, physical appearance, or childhood. They are in this world to repair contrasts and make them feel right, prepared to give their life for a sibling or a companion. Gemini Love and Sex Fun and constantly prepared for a scholarly challenge, Gemini sees love first through correspondence and verbal contact, and discover it as significant as physical contact with their accomplice. At the point when these two consolidate, impediments all appear to blur. Curious and constantly prepared to be a tease, a Gemini could invest a great deal of time with various darlings until they locate the correct one who can coordinate their astuteness and vitality. They need fervor, assortment, and enthusiasm, and when they locate the opportune individual, a darling, a companion and somebody to converse with joined into one, they will be loyal and resolved to consistently cherish their heart.

Cancer

Profoundly instinctive and wistful, Cancer can be one of the most testing zodiac signs to become acquainted with. They are extremely passionate, delicate, and care profoundly about issues of the family and their home. Malignant growth is thoughtful and appended to individuals they keep close. Those brought into the world with their Sun in Cancer are extremely faithful and ready to understand other individuals' torment and enduring.

The indication of Cancer has a place with the component of Water, much the same as Scorpio and Pisces. Guided by feeling and their heart, they could experience serious difficulties mixing into their general surroundings. Being ruled by the Moon, periods of the lunar cycle develop their inner riddles and make short-lived passionate examples that are outside their ability to control. As kids, they need more adapting and guarded systems for the external world and must be drawn closer with consideration and comprehension, for that is the thing that they give consequently.

Absence of persistence or even love will show through emotional episodes sometime down the road, and even narrow-mindedness, self-centeredness or control. They rush to help other people, similarly as they rush to keep away from strife, and once in a while advantage from the close battle of any sort, continually hitting somebody more grounded, greater, or more dominant than they envisioned. When content with their life decisions, Cancer agents will be glad and substance to be encompassed by a cherishing family and amicability in their home.

Enthusiasm can cause them to imperil their very own prosperity, battling for another person's motivation as though others can turn into their higher power. The Crab realizes where they're going, however, this is frequently off course, at any rate until they gain proficiency with their exercises and start depending entirely on themselves.

Leo

Individuals brought into the world under the indication of Leo are normal conceived pioneers. They are sensational, inventive, fearless, predominant and amazingly hard to oppose, ready to accomplish anything they need to in any everyday issue they focus on. There is a particular solidarity to a Leo and their "ruler of the wilderness" status. Leo frequently has numerous companions for they are liberal and faithful. Self-assured and alluring, this is a Sun sign equipped for joining various gatherings of individuals and driving them as one towards a common reason, and their solid comical inclination makes cooperation with other individuals considerably simpler.

Leo has a place with the component of Fire, much the same as Aries and Sagittarius. This makes them caring, in adoration with life, attempting to snicker and have a decent time. Ready to utilize their brain to tackle even the most troublesome issues, they will effectively step up to the plate in settling different confused circumstances. Led by the Sun, Leo adores this red-hot substance in the sky, truly just as figuratively. They are in a quest for mindfulness and consistent development of inner self. Mindful of their wants and character, they can without much of a stretch request all that they need, however, they could simply unwittingly disregard the necessities of other individuals in their pursuit for individual addition or status. At the point when a Leo delegate turns out to be too affectionate and connected to their accomplishments and how other individuals see them, they become an obvious objective, fit to be brought down.

The Lion consistently talks about fortitude. This is a creature dauntless and difficult to challenge, hurt or demolish, their lone shortcomings being trepidation and hostility towards those they go up against. Notwithstanding, they ought to never remain there for long. With their head high, they need to confront others with poise and regard, failing to raise a voice, a hand, or a weapon, valiantly strolling through the woods they rule.

Virgo

Virgos are continually focusing on the littlest subtleties and their profound feeling of mankind makes them one of the most cautious indications of the zodiac. Their efficient way to deal with life guarantees that nothing remains to risk, and in spite of the fact that they are regularly delicate, their hearts may be shut for the external world. This is a sign regularly misjudged, not on the grounds that they do not have the capacity to express, but since they won't acknowledge their sentiments as substantial, genuine, or even applicable when contradicted to reason.

Virgo is an Earth sign, fitting consummately between Taurus and Capricorn. This will prompt a solid character, however one that favors traditionalist, efficient things and a great deal of reasonableness in their regular day to day existence. These people have a sorted out life, and in any event, when they let go of tumult, their objectives dreams still have carefully characterized fringes in their psyches. Always stressed that they missed a detail that will be difficult to fix, they can stall out in subtleties, ending up excessively basic and worried about issues that no one else appears to think much about.

Since Mercury is the decision planet of this sign, its agents have a well-created feeling of discourse and composing, just like every other type of correspondence. Numerous Virgos may seek after a profession as scholars, columnists, and typists, however their need to serve others makes them feel great as parental figures, on reasonable assistance.

Libra

Individuals brought into the world under the indication of Libra are quiet, reasonable, and they abhor being distant from everyone else. Association is significant for them, as their mirror and somebody enabling them to be simply the mirror. These people are entranced by equalization and balance, they are in a consistent pursue equity and balance, acknowledging through life that the main thing that ought to be really imperative to themselves in their own internal character. This is somebody prepared to do about anything to stay away from struggle, keeping the harmony at whatever point conceivable

Libra is one speck of parity in the ocean of various limits, showed uniquely through the fifteenth level of this superb sign, an article among creatures and individuals. There is something dreadfully uncertain about Libra as though they were uncertain which plate to trouble straightaway, mindful that things pass and instruct us to be cautious around other individuals. Whatever we do in our lifetimes, just serves to point the route for our Souls towards that "higher power" to at last measure our reality. Disclosing to us where we turned out badly or what we did well, Libras unwittingly instruct us that genuine freedom covers up in daintiness.

Scorpio

Scorpio-conceived are enthusiastic and self-assured individuals. They are resolved and conclusive, and will research until they discover reality. Scorpio is an incredible pioneer, constantly mindful of the circumstance and furthermore includes conspicuously in creativity.

Scorpio is a Water sign and lives to involvement and express feelings. In spite of the fact that feelings are significant for Scorpio, they show them uniquely in contrast to other water signs. Regardless, you can be certain that the Scorpio will stay discreet, whatever they might be.

Pluto is the planet of change and recovery, and furthermore the ruler of this zodiac sign. Scorpios are known by their quiet and cool conduct, and by their puzzling appearance. Individuals regularly state that Scorpio-conceived are furious, most likely on the grounds that they see very well the standards of the universe. Some Scorpio-conceived can look more established than they really are. They are fantastic pioneers since they are devoted to what they do. Scorpios loathe untruthfulness and they can be extremely desirous and suspicious, so they have to figure out how to adjust all the more effectively to various human practices. Scorpios are daring and, in this way, they have a ton of companions.

Sagittarius

Inquisitive and vigorous, Sagittarius is perhaps the greatest voyager among all zodiac signs. Their receptive outlook and philosophical view spur them to meander the world over looking for the significance of life. Sagittarius is a social butterfly, idealistic and energetic, and preferences changes. Sagittarius-brought into the world can change their musings into solid activities and they will effectively accomplish their objectives.

Like the other fire signs, Sagittarius should be continually in contact with the world to encounter however much as could be expected. The decision planet of Sagittarius is Jupiter, the biggest planet of the zodiac. Their eagerness has no limits, and in this way, individuals brought into the world under the Sagittarius sign have an incredible comical inclination and a serious interest.

Opportunity is their most prominent fortune in light of the fact that at exactly that point they can unreservedly travel and investigate various societies and methods of reasoning. In light of their trustworthiness, Sagittarius-conceived are regularly anxious and unseemly when they have to state or accomplish something, so it's imperative to figure out how to convey what needs to be in a tolerant and socially adequate manner.

Capricorn

Capricorn is an indication that speaks to time and obligation, and its agents are customary and frequently intense naturally. These people have an inward condition of autonomy that empowers huge advancement both in their own and expert lives. They are bosses of discretion and can lead the way, make strong and practical plans, and oversee numerous individuals who work for them whenever. They will gain from their mix-ups and get to the top dependent on their experience and mastery.

Having a place with the component of Earth, similar to Taurus and Virgo, this is the last sign in the trio of common sense and establishing. In addition to the fact that they focus on the material world, however, they can utilize the most out of it. Lamentably, this component additionally makes them hardened and now and again too difficult to even think about moving from one viewpoint or point in a relationship. They experience considerable difficulties tolerating contrasts of other individuals that are excessively a long way from their character, and out of dread may attempt to force their customary qualities forcefully.

Saturn is the decision planet of Capricorn, and this planet speaks to limitations of numerous types. Its impact makes these individuals reasonable and mindful, yet in addition chilly, far off and unforgiving, inclined to the sentiment of blame and went to the past. They have to figure out how to excuse so as to make their very own life lighter and increasingly positive.

Continuously prepared to change into something that drives those frightening things away, Capricorn talks about every regular chain response of dread, where one alarming thing prompts numerous others, ascending as guarded instruments that lone exacerbate the situation. Drenched in their mystery, they face the world similarly as they are – bold enough to never flee, however always scared of their inward beasts.

Aquarius

Aquarius-conceived are modest and calm, yet then again they can be whimsical and fiery. Be that as it may, in the two cases, they are profound scholars and exceptionally educated individuals who love helping other people. They can see without bias, on the two sides, which makes them individuals who can undoubtedly tackle issues.

Despite the fact that they can without much of a stretch adjust to the vitality that encompasses them, Aquarius-conceived have a profound should be some time alone and away from everything, so as to reestablish control. Individuals brought into the world under the Aquarius sign, take a gander at the world as a spot brimming with potential outcomes. Aquarius is an air sign, and thusly, utilizes his brain at each chance. On the off chance that there is no psychological incitement, they are exhausted and come up short on inspiration to accomplish the best outcome.

The decision planet of Aquarius, Uranus has a meek, unexpected and now and again forceful nature, however, it likewise gives Aquarius visionary quality. They are fit for seeing the future and they know precisely what they need to do five or quite a while from now.

Uranus additionally gave them the intensity of snappy and simple change, so they are known as masterminds, progressives, and humanists. They feel great in a gathering or a network, so they continually endeavor to be encompassed by other individuals.

The most concerning issue for Aquarius-conceived is the inclination that they are restricted or obliged. On account of the craving for opportunity and equity for all, they will consistently endeavor to guarantee the right to speak freely of discourse and development. Aquarius-conceived have a notoriety for being cold and inhumane people, yet this is only their protection component against untimely closeness. They have to figure out how to confide in others and express their feelings in a sound manner.

Pisces

Pisces are neighborly, so they regularly end up in an organization of altogether different individuals. Pisces are magnanimous. They are continually ready to help other people, without wanting to get anything back. Pisces is a Water sign and all things considered this zodiac sign is described by sympathy and communicated enthusiastic limit.

Their decision planet is Neptune, so Pisces are more natural than others and have an imaginative ability. Neptune is associated with music, so Pisces uncover music inclinations in the most punctual phases of life. They are liberal, humane and incredibly dependable and minding. Individuals brought into the world under the Pisces sign have an instinctive comprehension of the existence cycle and in this way accomplish the best enthusiastic association with different creatures.

Pisces-conceived are known by their intelligence, yet affected by Uranus, Pisces now and then can play the job of a saint, so as to grab the eye. Pisces are rarely judgmental and continually sympathetic. They are likewise known to be most tolerant of all the zodiac signs.

Chapter 3

Getting To Know The Planets

Crystal gazing is about the Sun, the Moon, and the nine planets—these are at the very heart of soothsaying, both old and current. We as a whole know some cosmology, just by having seen the Sun and the Moon in the sky, and the vast majority of us have presumably observed Venus, and considerably Jupiter, more than once; however what we need to realize here is something other than the galactic estimation of these bodies, we need to know their prophetic worth. What do these bodies mean in our natal outlines?

The cutting edge celestial prophet realizes that planets don't make things occur here on Earth. We watch the perpetual planetary examples framing and dissolving in the sky, much as we see planes composing smoke letters over the sky, and we attempt to peruse that composition. What's going on out there in space and what's going on down here on earth are both occurring in a similar minute and a similar general space. Something very similar is going on all over, and there are simply various methods for communicating it. Crystal gazers figure out how to peruse the language of the planets and the stars so they can all the more likely comprehend what's going on here on Earth. The key players in this are the Sun, the Moon, and the Planets.

Maybe the most significant first idea to note is that those bodies out there are not simply detached substances. They work and drape all together—the nearby planetary group. What's more, they have all been doing this for an extremely lengthy timespan, so they have discovered the perfect separations to keep, one from another, as they all circle around the Sun. This incorporated adjusted framework is more seasoned than whenever we can quantify and will presumably last longer than whenever we can envision. Now ever, this whole framework has settled down and discovered its very own special musicality and pace.

Where we sit, on Earth, there are two planets inside Earth's circle, Mercury and Venus, and various planets outside of that circle: Mars, Jupiter, Saturn, and so forth. Step by step, over recorded time, every one of these incredible wonderful bodies has drawn around it a huge measure of legend and importance. These are not only a lot of rocks revolving around the Sun. There is increasingly more proof that our whole close planetary system, yet our whole universe, is an intelligible framework that some way or another imparts inside itself, at any rate, conveys enough data to keep on staying flawless—lucid.

Maybe your presentation, up until now, to this legend and convention, adds up to minimal more than what you have heard individuals state, possibly things, for example, "It's Mercury retrograde, so don't sign that agreement," or, "Host your gathering at the Full Moon, that is the point at which the vitality is high." What we need to do here is set aside the effort to truly become acquainted with the planets and what they need to state to us.

The Lights

The two most significant bodies are the Sun and the Moon, and, throughout the entire existence of soothsaying, this pair, together, is classified "The Lights." One light sparkles and the different reflects. You can't look legitimately into the Sun, yet you can, pretty much, discover your way around in obscurity by the reflected light of the Moon—by evening glow. What's more, the Sun isn't simply one more body in the nearby planetary group; it is the body around which the majority of the others rotate—the very heart and focal point of the close planetary system. The Sun is, most importantly, the most significant body in the entire framework, cosmically; yet, in addition prophetically. There is no correlation.

Along these lines, the Moon is the second most significant glorious body, not on the grounds that it has any mass or significance outside of how it impacts earth, but since it is about the main way we can get light from the Sun other than from the Sun itself. We as a whole take a gander at the Moon—we can't investigate the Sun. Since the commencement of soothsaying, much has been made of the way that the Moon transports to and fro between the space past the world's circle and the space inside that circle. It has been said that it continuously bolsters us the light of the Sun, by degrees, with the goal that we can acclimatize it into our lives—rather like an extraordinary mother supporting us. What's more, the Moon is loaded up with puzzles. The Mysteries of the Moon have been a basic piece of mysterious legend for a very long time. We can get into a portion of that later, however, for the time being, how about we turn out a portion of the more typical watchwords and general portrayals of the Sun and the Moon.

The Sun

The Sun isn't a planet, yet one of the Lights, and it is critical to us all. It is the wellspring of all light warmth and life, and the center around which the whole nearby group of planets rotate. In soothsaying, the Sun has consistently represented the Self, with a capital "S." It has an inseparable tie to what we endeavor to find, what we would like to move toward becoming, and what we treasure in mature age. It is a definitive reference point. The Sun is the whole procedure of life. Maybe everything that could possibly be said is: The Sun is Shining.

The Moon

The Moon, not by any means a planet, is the guardian of Earth. She invests her energy carrying from within the world's circle to the outside, and back. The Moon mirrors the light of the Sun as would an extraordinary mirror, illuminating the evening of our lives, interminably redistributing the sun-powered light all through her stages. She is the extraordinary mother, the nurturer, and the belly from which all life emerges. The Moon holds numerous riddles, some of which we will go into in another area. By the Sun, the Moon is the most significant body in the sky for us.

Other External Planets

At any rate, from where we sit on Earth, there are planets within the world's circle (Mercury and Venus), and planets past the world's circle (Mars, Jupiter, and Saturn). What's more, past this, we have the purported external or supernatural planets—Uranus, Neptune, and Pluto—which we will contemplate later. Since we live here on Earth, we can look either internal toward the Sun, at the planets Mercury and Venus, the inward planets (obscurely, these planets are a piece of our inward life, as we have called attention to) or we can look outside ourselves, to the planets Mars, Jupiter, and Saturn. These are outer or outside our skin. How about we start with these last three planets; the very request of them—Mars, Jupiter, Saturn—as they exist outside the circle of the earth, is significant, and discloses to us something. How about we go over these planets quickly, figuring out them.

We have various areas on the understanding of the planets incorporated into this course, so you can search for one that best suits you. Here are clear short depictions.

Mercury

Mercury signifies communication of all forms. This includes thoughts, ideas, and words—all of which may be spoken or written gossip, messages, and news. These spin off to deeds, paperwork, letters, documents and papers, in general; also, schooling, logic, reason, and all mental processes.

Venus

Venus signifies possessions, acquisitions, and money; thus, this planet also pertains to jewelry, decorative items, museums, various designs, and art in the general sense. It may also indicate younger women. This can either be a sweetheart or mistress.

Mars

Mars signifies force. As a result, this planet pertains to hunters, adventurers, weapons, the police force, and soldiers. This also includes athletes, sports, and exercise. You can also involve violence, crime, war, combat, and enemies when discussing this planet.

Jupiter

Jupiter has something to do with succession, success, and any simple continuance. This pertains to how people manage to provide continuity in life. The Hindu word for Jupiter is Guru, which tells us a lot. This planet is considered as our guide, our teacher. It shows us the ways to get through this life. Path or success in any career as Jupiter indicates our calling or vocation and career. This also includes how we solve the problems that life decides to throw at us.

Saturn

Saturn signifies confines, boundaries, restraints, and limits. Thus, this planet involves the imagery of teeth, property, skeletons, foundations, buildings, and more. Also, this planet considers organizations, corporations, time, laws, and rules.

Uranus

Uranus signifies discoveries, inventions, patents, electricity, computers, insight, innovation, technology, and more. Also, it pertains to revolution, freedom, and rebellion. Moreover, imageries like lightning, earthquake, accidents, divorce, sudden events, and separation are associated with this planet.

Neptune

Neptune signifies embracement, compassion, cherishing, union, unity, oceans, seas, and other bodies of water. Also, this planet pertains to film, images, movies, photography, and music, as well as alcohol, hallucinations, and an escape.

Pluto

Pluto signifies extreme sensitivity and vulnerability, transformation, and any deep change. This also pertains to all things buried and hidden, the occult, detectives, investigations, big business, and power politics.

Chapter 4

The Horoscope Diagram

What is the Horoscope Diagram?

They state individuals don't accompany a guidance manual. We tend to disagree! Your crystal gazing outline holds the way into your character and way. A crystal gazing birth outline—additionally called a soothsaying natal graph or the horoscope chart—is a guide of where every one of the planets was in their voyage around the Sun (from our vantage point on earth) at the definite minute you were conceived. A soothsaying outline perusing can uncover your qualities and shortcomings, your chances for soul development, the best planning for your most significant moves.

To compute your crystal gazing birth outline, you'll need your time, date and spot of birth. A few people don't have the foggiest idea about their introduction to the world time. In the event that you can't discover it on your introduction to the world declaration, you can have a go at reaching the Vital Records office in your state or region of birth. Furthermore, if that still doesn't work, make as close of a gauge as you can or enter 12:00 early afternoon. Without a birth time, you won't have the option to precisely become familiar with your rising sign, or ascendant. Nor will you effectively realize which houses the planets in your outline fall in. However, there is still a LOT of information you can gather by entering your date and area of birth—so don't let that prevent you from looking at your soothsaying natal diagram.

What can an astrologer find in your diagram?

Soothsaying outlines can turn up an amazing understanding of your examples and inclinations. They're a phenomenal method for comprehension of your own "vulnerable sides" and utilizing that learning for self-awareness and personal development. You can realize which gifts to create and where you may have shaky areas to create.

Ordinarily, a soothsayer searches for a couple of key things in the birth diagram:

- What zodiac sign and which of the 12 houses every planet in the outline is in.
- Venus, Mars and the moon's zodiac sign and house for affection.
- Saturn for where you may need to work more diligently, Jupiter for where you could be fortunate.
- The "viewpoints" or edges framed between any two planets.
- In the event that there's a "stellium" (at least 3 planets in a single sign), which makes an overwhelming convergence of one explicit vitality for the individual.
- The equalization of components (planets in the fire, earth, air, and water signs) in the diagram.
- The equalization of characteristics in the diagram (planets in cardinal, alterable or fixed signs).
- The pattern framed by the planets (there are 7 traditional diagrams "shapes").

A celestial prophet will include the components and characteristics and "score" the diagram. On the off chance that there's an absence of one quality or power of another, they'll exhort the customer on the best way to for all intents and purposes bring more balance into their lives. We call this Astro-Ayurveda since it's the specialty of adjusting your graph!

74

There are multiple times when it's particularly productive to investigate your soothsaying graph: toward the start of consistently and on your birthday. For the New Year, we'd recommend doing what's known as a travel graph (additionally called a "natal in addition to travels" outline). This may require the direction of an expert soothsayer on the grounds that the understanding work can get perplexing! For this situation, you start with your own natal (birth) outline, and contrast it with the traveling (moving) planets, i.e., the present places of the planets in the sky.

What different sorts of crystal gazing outlines are there?

Solar Return Charts: Also known as your "birthday outline," the sun-powered return graph gives you a one-year diagram that keeps going from your present birthday until your next one. These outlines will shift contingent upon area. Adjust your festivals to the stars for the best outcomes!

Compatibility Astrology Charts: notwithstanding the soothsaying birth outline, you can do a crystal gazing similarity graph to perceive how you'll coexist with other individuals. You can cast two sorts of similarity graphs. A synastry graph looks into the planets in your diagram and the other person's. Composite outline midpoints your two graphs utilizing a "midpoint technique." It makes a solitary, mixed diagram that uncovers the quintessence of your relationship. A composite graph regards your relationship as though it was its very own substance or a third "individual" (which from multiple points of view is valid!).

Astrology Charts for Planning Events: You can do diagrams for individuals and furthermore for occasions. Simply invest the effort, date, and area of the occasion being referred to and you can cast a crystal gazing graph for it. For instance, in case you're arranging a gathering or a major pitch meeting, you can enter the time, date and area to perceive how the stars adjust.

Shouldn't something be said about Vedic crystal gazing graphs?

The Western soothsaying diagram is portrayed as a wheel isolated into 12 distinct fragments, or houses. It goes back to You can do a Vedic soothsaying outline (or Jyotish crystal gazing graph) or a Chinese crystal gazing diagram, which will ascertain the information in an unexpected way.

To what extent have these sorts of soothsaying diagrams been near?

At Astrostyle, we work with the Western crystal gazing framework, which goes back a great many years. People have followed the development of the sky since human advancement unfolded. As far back as 6000 B.C., the Sumerians noticed the voyages of planets and stars. Around 3300 B.C. the Babylonians (otherwise called the Chaldeans) started developing what the Sumerians began, building up the primary mysterious framework for more than a huge number of years. They made the zodiac wheel that we use today (with planets and houses) around 700 B.C. The most seasoned realized horoscope outline is accepted to date to 409 B.C.

Chapter 5

Personality Analysis Using Psychological Astrology

Crystal gazing can edify our conduct and explain relationships throughout everyday life. Nonetheless, it can't and shouldn't bind an individual. A celestial birth picture comprises of images that have been converted into words and solid models in the accompanying content.

When understanding them, you will find inconsistencies. For instance, one segment portrays the requirement for a quiet and stable relationship, and another area says that you need incitement and assortment inside a relationship. Such a logical inconsistency contains the requesting challenge to express the two alternate extremes. The accompanying content isn't a "fortune-telling horoscope" since only you are the modeler of your predetermination. The horoscope depicts the "crude material" that you have accessible.

Ascendant in Capricorn

With the ascendant in Capricorn, you establish a dependable and genuine connection. You seek security and acknowledge progressive systems. Individuals believe you to be somebody who pays attention to life, making progress toward objectives in a restrained and mindful way.

Sun in Libra

In your deepest being, you take a stab at equity, agreement, and harmony. Your prudent and approachable way gives you a chance to be prevalent with numerous individuals. Disposing of contentions is one of your worries. In doing as such, you can create extensive discretionary capacities in the event that you face the contention and don't just accommodate for harmony. You are great at moving toward other individuals. Simultaneously, you generally underscore what you share for all intents and purpose and what interfaces you with them. You frequently give too little consideration to the distinctions.

Sun in the Ninth House

You might want to genuinely apply the characteristics depicted above and along these lines extend your own frame of reference. Framing conclusions, issues concerning theory and training, and outside societies, just as the trade with individuals who think contrastingly and are critical to you, similar to the probability of persuading others regarding your feelings.

Moon in Leo

Your forces of the creative mind are very enthusiastic. You consider each to be a circumstance as a component of a more prominent setting and respond in like manner with emotional signals. With your regular warmth, you can be extremely winning. Since you esteem consideration, you will in general now and again place yourself a lot at the focal point of consideration.

Moon in the Seventh House

You have an incredible requirement for being as one and feel increasingly comprehensive when you are seeing someone. Your interceding way should make it simple for you to build up contacts. You endeavor to adjust and underline what you share practically speaking with others and what associates you with them. On the off chance that you react an excessive amount to other individuals, you will experience issues in inclination your own needs.

Mercury in Libra

You are a representative and don't care for transparently defying someone else in a discussion. With respect and natural seeing, for all intents and purposes in a hidden way, you endeavor to tell another person your supposition. At the point when you are engaged with a discussion with somebody, you stress what you share practically speaking; you want to dismiss contrasts.

Mercury in the Ninth House

You need to share your contemplations and learning. With your scholarly and verbal capacities, you might want to rouse and persuade others. Along these lines, you are presumably fit for functioning as an instructor, teacher, or sales representative.

Venus in Virgo

Excellence is intently connected with handy contemplations for you. Wonderful things that are just there to satisfy the eye effectively motivation you to address whether they merit spending the cash on them. Delightful things ought to likewise satisfy a reason. Then again, you have certain tasteful measures for the articles of day by day use, making both a down to earth and delightful condition for yourself.

Venus in the Eighth House

You don't have a lot of enthusiasm for a shallow relationship. You need to have energy and sexuality and furthermore live it out. At the point when you go into an association, you request an absolute commitment from your accomplice; one could nearly say that you need to have the person in question. You have a sharp eye for what is covered and covered up in an organization. You need to test your accomplice's dull sides. On the off chance that your accomplice has a past that you don't think about, you will scarcely disregard the person in question until you know it all.

Mars in Gemini

Most importantly, you stand up for yourself by utilizing words. Correspondence is a method for you to make things occur; it could nearly be known as a weapon for your situation. You rationally create fight plans and use them to intentionally advocate for yourself in discussions. You acknowledge vivacious dialogs and can likewise contend when you get irritated.

Mars in the Sixth House

With extraordinary likelihood, the sort of man who captivates you exemplifies huge numbers of these characteristics. This implies you like down to earth, reasonable, and reasonable men with whom you can ace regular day to day existence and achieve an occupation. An adoration relationship that additionally empowers you to fill in as a group ought to especially speak to you.

Jupiter in the Seventh House

You like having your accomplice bolster you since this makes it workable for you to show yourself as liberal and hopeful. You bring a significant inclination to venture into a relationship, which isn't constantly good with the social ideas of organization and marriage. You will, in general, take a gander at an organization from the light side and show little ability to chip away at common issues together.

Saturn in the Sixth House

Fundamentally, your assignment is to accept accountability for your reality, which means for your day-by-day life, your body, and your wellbeing. This doesn't imply that you must be impeccable. Maybe you can likewise force yourself to assign certain undertakings and along these lines decrease the weight and requests without anyone else execution.

Uranus in the Fifth House

You look for conceivable outcomes for articulation that don't relate to the standard. Do you like to play-act? You enjoy changing yourself. You appreciate more than once showing yourself in an alternate getup. You are inventive and have the inclination to show yourself off.

Neptune in the Eighth House

It is hard for you to effectively evaluate social qualities and power structures. On the off chance that you manage acquired cash or different qualities that have been endowed to you, you may effortlessly believe this to be a typical property. It might potentially go through your hands.

Pluto in the Seventh House

"Win big or bust!" is your witticism seeing someone. Your accomplice needs to have you totally - or you need that person totally - with body, brain, and soul. Your connections are serious and energetic. This likely additionally incorporates the dread of being left and the endeavor to control and control the relationship and the accomplice. An affection relationship without power games, without testing each other's quality, without energy, and without envy resembles a soup without salt for you.

Chapter 6

What You Need To Know About Numerology

Numerology is a representative investigation of musicality, cycles, and vibration. The careful birthplace of numerology is discretely covered in the fogs of time. If one somehow managed to be definite, it could be said the numerology has its birthplace before the very beginning! In its most obscure structure numerology essentially mirrors the tides and cycles of creation as set moving by the Creator.

It is identified with crystal gazing, a superior known cousin of emblematic examination. They are both worried about the relationship of edges and vibrations coming about because of the exercises of heavenly developments and the cycles of time, space and the continuous procedure of advancement.

The investigation of numerology started with man's most punctual endeavor to comprehend the connection between self and the universe. In written history, it is realized that numbers were noteworthy in the Sanskrit of the antiquated Hindu culture, just as in old China. Current numerology, in its advancement, was likewise affected by the Arabic arrangement of numbers. One more significant branch is in the convention and imagery of the Kaballa. The Orient likewise has a rich convention of offering an incentive to numbers. The Bible is also weighed down with a significant history of imagery dependent on numbers. Inside the historical backdrop of these societies is an abundance of yet unfamiliar insight dependent on the recondite lessons of their numerical customs.

The individual most answerable for affecting the technique for numerology being used today was Pythagoras, a Greek thinker conceived between around 600 and 590 BC. Pythagoras established a school where the guidance of science, music, space science, and reasoning was directed related to elusive intelligence. He showed the connection between man and the celestial laws as reflected in the arithmetic of numbers. Upon his philosophical quality and numerical commitments the investigation of numerology, as it is today, has been set up.

There were said to have been two degrees of lessons inside the school: the exoteric and the exclusive. Today huge numbers of those understudies of old still exercise their enthusiasm for numbers. The exoteric understudies slant toward arithmetic and science and frequently have next to zero respect for the natural side of numbers (numerology). The elusive understudies in this day and age can be discovered working with numerology and in some cases exceptionally progressed and hypothetical arithmetic. These previous exclusive understudies, generally, experience difficulty learning standard scientific educating. Inquisitively, you discover bookkeepers and accountants who have worked with numbers for quite a long time and all of a sudden become entranced with numerology.

The present researchers and technologists are giving regularly expanding consideration to the utilization of vibrations and frequencies. The approach of power presented different utilizations of working with common cycles. Radio, TV, x-beams, and sub-nuclear cycles are a few aspects of present-day innovation that have opened the entryway to more noteworthy investigation and use of the standards of repeating motions. The new learning of the biorhythm

83

cycles has made the open increasingly proficient about exactly that it is so critical to know about the repetitive examples in our day-by-day life.

Physicists have discovered that materials recently characterized as idle, likewise have their very own awareness, which is built up by their pace of vibration or recurrence. The advances in quantum material science and astronomy teem with heightening revelations about our universe and our relationship to it. Additional comprehension of the GUT (Grand Unified Theory) is distributed day by day. The investigation of numerology has from its origination held the way to understanding the GUT. Maybe increasingly significant numerology holds a vital aspect for encountering it directly. The investigation of numerology can take you from an onlooker of the occasion of advancement to a cognizant member in it.

Numerology, as it is more regularly rehearsed, gives methods for understanding repetitive examples or characteristics related explicitly to the person's close to home life. By understanding one's specific beat, it ends up simpler to stream with life. With such understanding, one can turn into the ace of destiny, as opposed to a casualty of fate's conditions. Its application might be increasingly significant today during a time of uncontrolled realism and existential emergency than it was with the antiquated searcher.

The authentic representation gave in this is, as a matter of fact, short and concise. Different past essayists regarding the matter have given more subtleties to the generally disapproved. The accentuation of this volume is upon the utilization of numerical information in the present time and place.

Chapter 7

What You Need To Know About Kundalini Rising

Kundalini is inert vitality accepted to be snaked at the base of the spine. Kundalini likewise alludes to an arrangement of reflection that is intended to discharge this vitality. At the point when individuals have a kundalini arousing more prana (chi) is held in and goes through their sensory system. It is said that yoga can unblock the vitality from the root chakra and let it travel up the spine to enable you to interface with your spirit and super cognizance. Yogi Bhajan began Kundalini Yoga in the West in the wake of turning into an ace at age 17 in India. This kind of yoga was initially called Raj or Laya yoga and was passed down starting with one master then onto the next.

At the point when individuals experience the purifying intensity of kundalini rising, they become heart-focused and develop. So the inquiry is, would our societies advance if more individuals stirred? We, people, contrast from every other species in our capacity to watch ourselves inside an evolving universe. We can consider what we have originated from and where we might go. We know social and authentic records impact the manner in which we live; we have turned out to be progressively mindful by gaining from our past experience. At this moment, we are getting to be multidimensional.

In any case, the male-centric innovative society compromises our planet. Numerous miracles in the event that we are losing our endurance impulses with individuals gliding around in mass trance pushing keys on the internet while dwelling in medicated, overweight bodies. The individuals who permit kundalini vitality to move in their bodies regularly haul out of the mass trance. What does the planetary-development speculation have to do with mass culture?

The appropriate response is, Everything! Enacted kundalini vitality is the wellspring of the endurance impulse. At the point when we feel this perfect life power ascending in our bodies, we discharge Eros into the trap of life. A large number of us have found that significant life cycles can be utilized to improve self-awareness. Our subsequent stage is to make the cognizant inception into more advanced perspectives into a social aim. For instance, the time has come to utilize this learning to direct our youngsters. For a large number of years up until as of late, human social orders started their youngsters to enable them to explore key life entries. Kids must understand these different parts of life while they are youthful; that is the thing that will move societies and the planet back to adjust.

As indicated by old Eastern shrewdness, the snake control kundalini is wound in the root chakra and ascends the spine to the head. The most recent research on cerebrum science proposes that natural discharge is in the mind. At that point, similarly as with every single human sensation, what is transmitted from the mind is felt in the body. In the event that the kundalini trigger is the cerebrum, at that point, our psychological evaluation of our own development is the most freeing approach to keenly think about ourselves. What we believe is conceivable will be the following phase of human advancement.

Around the world, body/mind healers work one-on-one and with gatherings in workshops to help a large number of us clear decisions that square mending. Eco-feminist, Earth-focused networks and stylized occasions at consecrated destinations with indigenous individuals are establishing another vitality structure. They help all to

86

remember us that we can live in harmony and agreement and experience bliss in our individual family units once more. Clearly, we didn't ascend the long stepping stool of development without an explanation! Every individual who assumes microcosmic liability for the widespread issue is a piece of the arrangement in the universe. It is important in the event that you eat naturally, sustain with generosity, and secure the trap of life. The visionary film Avatar is a propelled composition of along these lines of being.

How could we lose this? For the last 5,000 years, human inventiveness has been channeled into fights and into structure urban areas and domains. After some time, individuals came to accept that an enemy causes their problems. The better approach for intuition recommends we quit pointing the fault at the "other" to assume liability for what we are doing ourselves, an extraordinary move in critical thinking. Those of us who have accomplished this new viewpoint should be delicate with those still caught in accusing their issues of others since they don't realize how to quit passing judgment on others to accuse everybody except themselves for their issues.

Worldwide mindfulness is separating the confidence in the foes out there. Banking debacles caused individuals to understand that on the off chance that one comes up short, all come up short. We should seek ourselves for the start of the issues. Nowadays, many maintain a strategic distance from legislative issues dependent on control and control by finding significant approaches to help society through recuperating and social activity. The possibility that we make our own reality can be the wellspring of excruciating and profound divisions between political sorts and social reformers since the two gatherings neglect to incorporate the inward and external substances. Unexpectedly, numerous social transformers can see that how we think makes the outcomes in the surveys. Be that as it may, they abstain from looking at the substance of their own personalities since they once in a while seek after genuine individual mending to clear internal agony. They believe they don't possess energy for individual recuperating work since they should spare the world.

We have gone to a point where the battle in the external world has gone to an apex, powerfully and delightfully punctuated by a progression of seven squares between Uranus and Pluto during 2012-15. Uranus rules change and Pluto rules confused change; the squares are constraining everyone to process the outcomes of 5000 years of man-centric culture. However, the tempering strength of these Uranus-Pluto squares makes everything feel terrible!

Numerous indigenous functions and world social occasions from 1987 to 2012 depended on different readings of the Mayan Calendar just as antiquated predictions. Symphonious Convergence in August 1987 started this extraordinary stage, and now we are breaking into another world. The finish of this long cycle in 2012 discharged us to pick cognizant interest in different measurements, for example, in the Galactic Center. The researcher Terence McKenna once said we were being destroyed to a transformative jump by a divine cognizance coordinating planetary advancement. As we have been watching ourselves in the developmental stream, we are intrigued by creation stories and archeological disclosures. In any case, this is a risky time since male-prevailing monotheistic world religions oppose the possibility of the stirred human. This strain, so evident in the critical condition of world issues, implies we are at the hardest point. The man centric society can't keep on harming the world. We should actuate ladylike powers and utilize right-mind aptitudes to neutralize this unevenness.

Extraordinary power is accessible to people in their enacted ladylike nature, the innovative capability of all-encompassing cerebrum synchronization. At the point when our right-cerebrum instinct works working together with our exceptionally grown left-mind, we look for a peaceful and imaginative culture that can encourage the total advancement of cognizance. We will not be isolated by vain detachment when we realize we are not the slightest bit better than some other components or species.

The Mayan worldview is shamanic, that is, a culture that purposefully created synchronistic points of view, instinct, and multidimensional observations. Shamanic societies love the female as the wellspring of life; at that point male and female together make regard forever. Figuring out how to use kundalini vitality makes a balance in human social orders. It is the best approach to cause the mass actuation of shamanic powers that falsehood lethargic in our bodies. We are the sacrosanct fire. Truly, there is an incredible point of reference for that the change of the individual is at the center of an illuminated society. There are endless instances of old societies that existed in a condition of harmony and concordance for hundreds and even a large number of years dependent on this conviction. These societies have deserted aesthetic, composed, and archeological records of profoundly created shamanic procedures. Mayan and Egyptian societies flourish with such proof, and the Hopi individuals of the hallowed Four Corners district of the American Southwest still keep up a shamanic culture that is as of now a large number of years old. Going more remote back in time, we as a whole are slipped from the individuals of the Mother Goddess. Regardless we hold this profound memory of how to make and live on the planet in a tranquil, sound way. From 12,000 to around 3500 years prior, living was fundamentally quiet, as indicated by such extraordinary women's activist researchers as Marija Gimbutas, William Irwin Thompson, Gerda Lerner, Riane Eisler, and Mary

Settegast. Birthing and a feeling of everything originating from the female was at the focal point of this Goddess culture.

Current individuals hold not very many social recollections from before 12,000 years prior because of disturbances that nearly wrecked our planet, however, the Goddess culture goes route once more into the fogs of time. The fall of the Minoan culture 3500 years prior finished the primordial Goddess culture with the emission of a colossal spring of gushing lava on Santorini that tossed the Aegean bowl into a long dim age. Extraordinary dread of nature resulted in the West that in the long run prompted the ill-conceived notion that God made the world for generally male utilization. The presence of this long period of ancient times is a confident sign that we could make such a culture again by people binding together their objectives.

Conclusion

Thank for making it through to the end of *"Astrology: A Beginners Guide to Understand Yourself and Others through the 12 Zodiac Signs and Horoscopes for Spiritual Growth. Master your Destiny thanks to Numerology and Kundalini Rising (Soul Purpose)"*, let's hope that you were able to remember some of the key points in this book.

The situation of the planets at the hour of our introduction to the world causes us in recognizing the feeble or solid aspects of our life. Crystal gazing can assist us with understanding better the occasions of our past. Other than aiding in staying away from strains in conjugal connections, business, and expert issues, crystal gazing likewise helps in getting a charge out of good wellbeing, success and profound headway. With the assistance of crystal gazing, we can find what characteristics we look for in an accomplice and how to beat any contradiction since we will have a superior comprehension of various characters.

Horoscope can give us an understanding of the mentality and the attributes of individuals with whom we live. Along these lines, we can all the more likely adjust to one another's qualities and shortcomings and we can likewise keep away from clashes and decrease the negative outcomes of the distinctions in the characters.

Crystal gazing is an awesome science that empowers us to investigate what's to come. Crystal gazing can demonstrate what anticipates us later on, what energies lie ahead and when is the best time to make a move to achieve your objectives. Along these lines, if we have at any rate a fundamental sign of what anticipates us, we can settle on choices all the more effectively.

Numerous individuals accept that contemplating our prophetic diagram will reveal to us which signs we are good with. The examination of celestial diagrams of two people can decide their level of similarity, regardless of whether it comes to sentiment, business connections or companionships.

Nevertheless, we would like to request from you a review on Amazon regarding your experience with this book.

VAGUS NERVE

The ultimate guide to Vagus Nerve stimulation. Reduce and Prevent Anxiety, Depression and Chronic illness. Quit Smoking and Drinking for Elavate Yourself and Boost your Self Esteem

By
Maria Carter

Introduction

Stress and emotions are natural encounters our bodies are designed to cope and process. On a daily basis, we run through one emotion to the next, from happy to sad to angry to afraid, often without giving any question or attention to them for longer than a few minutes. But, with the increase of mental health disorders on the rise, you may question whether our bodies are actually designed to handle the high stress or traumatic events so many have struggled to overcome?

What can be more alarming is the additional health problems that arise from what are typically considered mood or emotional disorders. While many types of therapies address the thoughts and feelings that cause emotional stress and medication help manage symptoms of the physical health condition, what seems to be overlooked is what actually connects mental disorders with physical complications?

These systems often directly or indirectly connect and have an impact on one another. The brain, heart, lungs, and digestive system, for instance, are all connected by one nerve. It is the heart of the brain-body connection. It is this nerve that can be the common link between mental health disorders and other physical health conditions.

Individuals who suffer from depression, autism spectrum disorder, chronic illnesses, and trauma struggle on a daily basis to find relief from their symptoms. While therapy can provide them with coping mechanisms, they still often have difficulty maintaining a healthy and peaceful state of mind. This book is designed to help those individuals who struggle with some of these common disorders. It can also provide valuable information to those who want to prevent and avoid these conditions and other physical health problems.

In this book, you will learn the inner workings of the body's complex autonomic nervous system. This system is responsible for regulating mood, emotions, heart rate, digestion, speech, hearing, and more. It is in this system you learn about the vagus nerve; the nerve that links the brain with the rest of the body and directly impacts how stress and emotions affect the proper function of vital organs.

You will find specific exercises, activities, and tips that can help you strengthen this nerve to combat depression, anxiety, PTSD, chronic illness, among others. While it is designed to provide hope, relief, and answers to those who suffer from mental or health disorder, it is a book that can positively impact all who read it. What you are about to learn is that our bodies have evolved to properly deal with any stress and/or emotions it newly encounters. We just haven't tuned in and learned how to properly use it to accomplish this.

While the vagus nerve functions naturally, age and other stress factors can inhibit its activity leading to a decreased vagal tone. This, therefore, means that we need to equip ourselves with the knowledge on how to stimulate and activate the vagus nerve in order to reap its self-healing benefits. Not only is the vagus nerve effective in the prevention of certain conditions, but it is also an effective therapy in the management of chronic inflammation and the resulting disorders such as rheumatoid arthritis.

This book is your guide to becoming more aware of the vagus nerve, finding out how it can help us, and learning more details about it. Let's get started!

Chapter 1

Vagus Nerve Fundamentals

What Is The Vagus Nerve?

The vagus nerve makes connects the brain and the majority of the body. Even if not directly connected, the vagus nerve also has a significant impact on the proper function and communication between other nerves, organs, and the brain.

It is also referred to as cranial nerve X, it is the longest-running cranial nerve going from the brain stem down to the colon. This is the most important cranial nerve as the communication superhighway between the brain and most of the body. It is at the heart of the autonomic systems.

The vagus nerve first extends from the very back of the brainstem, just before it meets the spinal cord. It extends out towards the jugular and down between the jugular vein and the internal carotid artery, which leads it on a path through the neck and chest and the abdomen. Along this line it sends information to most of the internal organs; it also has the responsibility of sending information to the brain in regards to how these organs are functioning.

Within the automatic nervous system, the brain is connected to the rest of the body, to all of those important parts that keep your body alive and functioning with impressive ease, through what is known as the vagus nerve.

The vagus nerve, simplified down, is a circuit of nerve cells that root throughout the body and brain—they go down to the body, interacting with the heart, lungs, and abdomen, and return back to the brain. This has one simple function—it allows the brain to communicate with those crucial parts. However, sometimes, that nerve circuit can malfunction, and when it does, there can be significant impacts on the individual. Just as how a car that has a dysfunctional electrical system may struggle to run effectively, the human body struggles when there are any errors in the vagus nerves. Ranging from deep breathing to yoga, there are a wide range of ways that you can regulate that nerve, and in doing so, you can find relief.

The vagus nerve is composed of almost 90% sensory fibers, which is why it is able to relate the condition of the internal organs clearly to the brain. It also has axons that go in and out of the medulla nuclei. There are four important intersections where this occurs:

- The dorsal nucleus—Responsible for sending signals from the parasympathetic nervous system to the intestines and other internal organs.
- The nucleus ambiguous—Sends a signal to the heart from the parasympathetic nervous system.
- The solitary nucleus—Receives information from the taste sensory system and makes connections to the internal organs.
- The spinal trigeminal nucleus—Responsible for organizing information from the outer ear, dura posterior cranial fossa, and the larynx. It interprets various levels of touch, pain, and temperature among these areas.

Your vagus nerve serves two main purposes. It handles both sensory functions and motor functions.

Motor functions require the vagus nerve to stimulate muscles so that they contract and move. This is most notable in the soft palate, larynx, heart, and digestive tract. Without this stimulation, your intestines wouldn't move and your stomach wouldn't process the food in it. You wouldn't be able to urinate, speak, or perform any number of other necessary functions. As you can see, this could be catastrophic if the vagus nerve isn't functioning completely.

A very quick and easy test to see if the vagus nerve is working adequately is to touch something soft to the back of the throat on either side. Most people will gag immediately. If you don't gag, this can signal an issue with the vagus nerve. Another option is to check the difference in heart rate when breathing in and when breathing out. The heart rate should return to normal almost immediately after breathing out. The gag reflex is an important one, since it helps people avoid choking.

Aside from reflexes, the vagus nerve keeps your breathing regular, speeding it up when needed, and regulates your heartbeat. If you are in danger, it stimulates adrenaline production and ensures that the body has the resources necessary to keep going when you need to fight or run.

The immune system, without the regulation of the vagus nerve, will cause an excess of inflammation, which results in autoimmune disease. Pain in joints, rashes on the skin, and hair falling out are just a few of the signs that things aren't working as they should. Fortunately, there is hope, even if your vagus nerve is damaged.

Longer than any other nerve in your autonomic nervous system, the vagus nerve wanders through the body. In fact, that is where it got its name—the name "vagus" comes directly from the Latin word for wandering. The nerve itself wanders through the body, allowing it to function normally when all is well with it. It regulates your body, allowing you to literally survive.

The nerve itself directly interacts with several parts of the body, namely the heart, lungs, and digestive tract. This makes the vagus nerve so incredibly important—it is involved in regulating the heart, breathing, and digestion.

When they do this, they are testing your vagus nerve, and so if you do not have a gag reflex when this not-so-fun part of your check up is happening, it may be an indicator that there is something wrong with your vagus nerve. This would then give the doctors somewhere to start with any treatments needing to be done, when they are looking for the root cause of your ailments. There is not a lot of point in treating symptoms if we can't get to the bottom of everything and fix the problem once and for all.

The vagus nerve is a large factor in the sensitivity of mucous membranes in the respiratory system and plays a massive role in transmitting the strength and rhythm of each breath you take as well as the frequency of your breaths. The vagus nerve also affects the larynx, esophagus, trachea, pharynx, as well as the bronchi, and will also assist with administering nerve fibers to the heart, pancreas, liver and last but not least, the stomach.

Nearly every part of the central body is affected by the vagus nerve. All those smaller nerve endings reach out to the neck and chest, as well as the abdomen. These nerves touch many organs, including the lungs, heart, intestines, stomach, and bladder, among others. Most people realize that the vagus nerve has an effect on things like the stomach and digestive tract, but they may not realize just how extensive it really is.

There have even been connections made between the types of food eaten and how the vagus nerve reacts. It can end up irritated and inflamed due to eating spicy food or alcohol. You can even end up with an inflamed vagus nerve when you're stressed out or anxious . . . which in turn can cause stress and anxiety.

It's all connected and the vagus nerve is the center of it all. When you manage your vagus nerve and keep it in good condition, your body parts will work in unison. That's the end goal, to ensure that your entire body is working, rather than treating just one part that is causing problems. Unfortunately, that's exactly what many doctors do, treat the individual problem. However, if one of your organs is not working properly, that is going to affect more organs and it's best to look at everything as a whole.

The location of this nerve is in the brainstem and travels all the way downwards. It starts at your brain, travels past the face and thorax, and all the way down to the abdomen. There are two sensory ganglia (which means two big pieces of nerve tissue that transmit the impulses) in this nerve.

Functions Of The Vagus Nerve

One of the greatest anomalies about the vagus nerve is that it is the major parasympathetic nerve of the entire body! This nerve is supplying parasympathetic fibers throughout the nervous system to all the most important organs of the body, especially focusing on those within the abdomen, chest cavity, neck and head. The vagus nerve is in charge of many of the body's main functions that all seem a bit strange to be linked together. The vagus nerve is also directly linked to your gag reflex when the back and sides of the throat are stimulated, it is linked to slowing your heart rate, and it can control your sweating and regulate your blood pressure. It can also stimulate peristalsis of the gastrointestinal tract as well as being able to control your vascular tone.

Our brain does not just react to external stimuli to keep our environment safe and conducive for us, it also requires constant communication with other body organs. Communication between the brain and other body organs serves to ensure the optimal functioning of the various body systems is maintained. Body organs require regulation such that processes can be activated or inhibited depending on the situation or physical state of our bodies.

If, for instance, you are jogging, your body will require more oxygen to facilitate the increased demand that is occasioned by physical activity. For this to happen, the heart and breathing rates need to increase, so that more air is pumped by the lungs and blood circulation is enhanced to increase the supply of this oxygen to the tissues and muscles. This ability of the body to regulate functions and maintain homeostasis is crucial for normal function and our overall health and wellbeing.

To accomplish body homeostasis, the vagus nerve functions in its parasympathetic role and inhibits the flight or fight responses initiated by the sympathetic nervous system in response to a threat or stressful situation. Let's say that you encounter a wild hog while out hiking in the woods. Once your brain registers the existence of this threat, your fight or flight responses will be instantly activated to enable you to either fight this threat or run away from it. All these responses are initiated to enable you to neutralize the threat and avoid possible harm.

Let's look at a different situation, where you have to do a public presentation and the idea of speaking in public is making you apprehensive and panicky. In this case, your body will activate the sympathetic responses of fight or flight to help you cope with this stress. Regardless of whether you are facing a physical threat or a perceived emotional threat, your sympathetic responses will not distinguish between physical and mental stresses and will react in the same way by initiating the fight or flight response.

The mode of action of the sympathetic responses of fight or flight is to basically increase the energy available to the body to enable it to fight or flee from a particular threat. This increase in energy is achieved by increasing your heart rate, which means blood is pumped at a faster rate and also increasing your respiration such that your breathing becomes quicker.

Now, imagine if you were constantly in a state of agitation as in the case of someone suffering from chronic stress, this would mean that your fight and flight response would be constantly activated. This means that you would have an accelerated heartbeat, increased rate of respiration, and inhibited digestive function for prolonged periods of time.

When the sympathetic system is not effectively counteracted by the parasympathetic system, the constant fight or flight responses will start to cause physical disorders by the overstimulation of certain functions. This is why the vagus nerve in its parasympathetic role in the nervous system is so important for optimum health. It ensures that the sympathetic responses are not active for prolonged periods of time unchecked.

The vagus nerve effectively puts the body back in a relaxed or rested state by slowing down the heartbeat, decreasing the rate of respiration, and stimulating digestive function. These interventions by the vagus nerve ensure that once a threat has been resolved, your body is reverted to a relaxed and rested state. This relaxed state is what creates a conducive environment for the body to engage its self-healing mechanism, prevents chronic inflammation, and mitigates against chronic stress and anxiety.

Without the effective functioning of the vagus nerve, the sympathetic nervous becomes overstimulated, and this, in turn, causes organ malfunction. To ensure that our vagal tone is high, there are measures we can take to routinely activate its parasympathetic effects and ensure that we reap the benefits of its self-healing power. We can activate the vagus nerve using various techniques such as meditation, exercise, breathing techniques, cold therapy, and many other techniques.

The vagus nerve has both sensory as well as motor functions that keep us ticking the way we should. Some of these functions include:

- The stimulation of muscles in the soft palate, which is in the roof of your mouth, as well as stimulating the larynx and pharynx inside your throat.
- Heart stimulation, which thereafter helps to lower your heart rate as well as regulate your blood pressure.
- The stimulation of the digestive tract in order to help you with digestion and passing your food through your system. This also includes stimulation of the esophagus.
- Stimulation of the sensitive skin behind your ears as a sensory piece, as well as sending information to the brain to trigger reflexes when stimulation is affecting the outer ear canal as well as the throat. You will also find that it plays a part in your taste sensations at the back of your mouth where the root of your tongue is.

When the vagus nerve gets stimulated very suddenly without any warning, you can cause a reaction called the vasovagal reflex to happen.

There are some people who are unfortunately prone to getting these reflexes although it is most commonly found due to stress, high amounts of pain, getting a sudden fright or even from a gastrointestinal problem from something you may have eaten that didn't quite agree with your insides.

When this vasovagal reflex does happen, it will cause your heart rate and blood pressure to drop very quickly, most often causing loss of consciousness or fainting. This is a condition that is called vasovagal syncope.

When the vagus nerve gets stimulated for therapeutic effects, you will find that you are able to have complete control over your body!

You can stimulate the vagus nerve to stop a nasty hiccup episode that is relentless, and doctors will often use the vagus nerve to help them diagnose a potential heart murmur or to treat depression.

In order for your brain to know the current status of what is happening to the organs around your body, it needs the signals from the vagus nerve to bounce back through those organs and send a sort of 'report' back to the brain in order to react further.

The vagus nerve has become so important in the medical industry that doctors are now finding that they can stimulate the vagus nerve using a device that gets placed in your chest, somewhat like a pacemaker, and send signals to the nerve through this device in order to get certain reactions from your body. Vagus nerve blocking is also fast becoming a popular method of treatment, especially aiding in weight loss as it has become far more superior to that of gastric bypass surgery!

Significance Of The Vagus Nerve

The wandering characteristic of the nerve enables it to send out information from the brainstem to body organs. Particularly, the nerve has full control of your parasympathetic nervous system, which is the central nerve. Besides, the nerve oversees numerous functions in the body as it enhances the communication of sensory and motor impulses to every organ. Vagus nerve regulates crucial aspects of human physiology, including digestion, sweating, blood pressure, and even speaking. It may be the missing link to achieve the treatment of incurable diseases that are characterized by inflammation and unconsciousness. The following are common ways in which the vagus nerve is significant to the human body:

Tackles Inflammation

It is reasonable to expect a certain degree of inflammation if you are injured or ill. However, prolonged inflammation may be upsetting and may hinder you from undertaking regular routines. Further, prolonged and recurring inflammation is a common symptom of chronic illnesses such as rheumatoid arthritis. Most of the time, people experience inflammation in their body organs, especially the joints and muscles, as they play a significant role in enabling you to carry on with day-to-day activities. To solve this issue, the vagus nerve has fibers that detect the presence of tumor necrosis factor (TNF), which indicates incipient inflammation. As a result, the nerve then alerts the brain, which produces the neurotransmitters responsible for fighting inflammation in the body. The neurotransmitters also assist the immune system in fighting the condition.

Controls The Heart

The electrical impulses from the vagus nerve acts as controllers of the heart. The natural muscle tissues set the pace at which the heart should pump the blood. However, the production of the acetylcholine chemicals slows the heart rate making you calm down, especially after a reaction to danger or attack. This association of the vagus nerve with the gastrointestinal tract communicates about the rate and amount of blood required during digestion and absorption of nutrients. The control of the heart rate plays a significant role in helping doctors determine the variability of your heart rate over a given timeframe. The information acquired in this test provides insights into the resilience of your vagus nerve and heart.

Relaxation

The ability and time to recover after injury, illness, and stress depend on the strength of your vagus response. To point out, the introduction of adrenaline and cortisol in your body helps in keeping you alert and reactive to immediate threats and dangers. On the other hand, the vagus nerve releases acetylcholine to calm your nerves and help release tension from your body. In this case, the tendrils present in the vagus nerve act as cables that reach all your body parts and organs to send instructions and signals. Most importantly, they counter the fight-or-flight response as they facilitate the creation of enzymes and proteins such as oxytocin, prolactin, and vasopressin that calm you down through regulation of the heart rate and the inhibition of stress reactors.

Connects Your Gut With The Brain

The gastrointestinal tract utilizes the vagus nerve to communicate to the brain. In most cases, electrical impulses in the nerve convey the feeling to the track making the feelings in your gut reach the brain quickly. Most of the abdominal organs depend on the vagus nerve to communicate with the brain. For instance, the parasympathetic innervation in the nerve utilizes branches in the stomach and the large colon to facilitate a smooth secretion and muscle contraction of these organs. Besides, the vagus nerve stimulates the production of acid and increases the rate of emptying in the stomach as you swallow food.

Weight Management

Communication in the gut-brain axis is facilitated by the vagus nerve. When the vagus nerve function is impaired, it loses the sensitivity that enables it to detect fullness in the stomach. When the vagus nerve cannot send a message to the brain that the stomach is full, it means you will not be able to know when you are full or not, and this is likely to cause overeating.

Stimulating the vagus nerve increases its sensitivity to the fullness signal from the stomach, and this increased sensitivity will cause you to feel fuller faster and, as such, will result in reduced food intake.

Stimulation Is A Medical Remedy

The use of electronic implants to stimulate the vagus nerve drastically reduces swelling and inflammation. A continued practice would result in remission of severe symptoms such as rheumatoid arthritis and save patients from toxic drugs in other acute conditions such as hemorrhagic shock. Sudden stimulation of the nerve lowers blood pressure through the production of the vasovagal reflex. Other medical conditions such as heart murmurs in dysautonomias still require excessive nerve stimulation to identify their origin and extent. Ultimately, advanced technology has improved how the vagus nerve is stimulated depending on the results desired. One of the most natural ways of vagal stimulation is the employment of the Valsalva maneuver. Nevertheless, other forms of stimulation, such as nerve-blocking, can only be used during the day and are known to facilitate weight loss.

Subsides Unconsciousness

If you feel queasy or treble whenever you get a flu shot or see blood, you are not weak. It might be a vagal syncope where your body overstimulates the vagus nerve as it responds to stress. In most cases, overstimulation of the vagus nerve drastically lowers your heart rate and, of course, the blood pressure. The slow flow of a small quantity of blood makes it only restricted to the brain where you are likely to lose consciousness. However, the condition is normalized by sitting or lying down.

A New Field Of Medicine

The discovery of how the vagus nerve influences body function makes it an essential asset in the medical profession. Specifically, the success of vagal nerve stimulation to treat epilepsy and inflammation has helped medics use electric impulses to treat health conditions using fewer or no medications and side effects. Again, the bioelectric study has emerged as the new class of medicine where electronics are implanted in the human body to fight symptoms and regulate nerve signals.

Good Memory

The vagus nerve has an immense contribution to your memory. A research that was conducted to test this with rats indicated that after the stimulation of their vagus nerve, they had increased memory. This is because of the neurotransmitter norepinephrine released by the activity into the amygdala, which preserved the memory. What is amazing is that further studies done in humans revealed that there was hope in the treatment of Alzheimer's disease.

Controls Your Heart Rate And Blood Pressure

We know that the vagus nerve is a wandering nerve. It may start from the brain, but it branches out to influence many organs and processes. One such organ is the heart.

It is wrong to say that the vagus nerve is directly connected to the heart. If that was the case, then we would suffer a cardiac arrest if the nerve sustained damage. Rather, the nerve is connected to the muscles that are connected to the heart. When the brain sends signals to the vagus nerve, it reacts to those signals and then transfers them over to the muscles near the heart. This, in turn, lets your heart know that it should slow down.

Enhances Your Breathing

The vagus nerve causes the neurotransmitter acetylcholine to inform your lungs that they need to breathe. There is a remedy used by people to curb different ailments cosmetically known as Botox. This has been seen to be dangerous to your body because it comes in and interrupts the production of acetylcholine. On the other hand, you can enhance and stimulate your vagus nerves by doing some breathing exercises. We shall be looking more on this further in the chapters.

Brings Out Your Gut Feeling

You have always heard that it is important to trust your gut feeling. Here is scientific proof that the gut feeling is right and real. There are electric impulses, which are also referred to as the action potential. Through this, your gut tells the vagus nerve to communicate to the brain about how you are feeling. Therefore, the brain takes action.

How The Vagus Nerve Manages It All

The vagus nerve provides a clear connection between the body and the brainstem. As a result, the brain monitors and remains aware of the functions throughout the body. The nerve also provides numerous features that contribute to other nerves within the body. If you wonder how a singular nerve could possess all that potential, you need to discover these characteristics:

Therefore, it efficiently provides the most extensive distribution of information. Comparatively, other smaller nerves would not reach the extent of the vagus nerve when it comes to swift body communication. The wandering characteristic also quickens the distribution of chemicals to prepare the body for reaction to the environment. It is an important aspect, especially if you are under attack or in danger, as the quick response allows you to take action while facing imminent danger within no time. Moreover, this character of the vagus nerve makes it acquire names that liken it to a separate life due to the number of organs that the nerve fibers are attached to. The attachment from the brain to the colon enables the nerve to coordinate the body functions or control them.

The vagus pair is located in the right and the left side of the human body and provides the skin with sensory and motor capabilities. The nerve covers a large portion of the human skin to enhance the sense of touch, which aids in feeling and understanding the surrounding. Besides, it ensures that the body is synchronized and up to date with how the body responds. Another key aspect is the uniform communication throughout the body ensuring that organs receive information simultaneously. This way, different body parts address the situation collectively.

Its access to critical organs. The vagus nerve manages all these functions and responsibilities through its capabilities and the fact that it is attached to some of the critical organs in your body. With excellent access to the heart, the nerve controls how the organ behaves in different situations. It is worth noting that your heart's behavior is a vital determinant of how you respond to safe or threatening situations. Generally, the vagus nerve has a parasympathetic nature that regulates how blood is pumped out of the heart. Most of the time, the heart will quickly pump when you are stressed or in need and will calm down once you are safe.

The connection created between the heart and the brain influences a unique combination and controls how your body reacts in some of these situations. Besides, the power of the nerve to the lungs enables breathing providing the body with sufficient oxygen and exhaling unwanted gases. Therefore, the vagus nerve remains vital for it is responsible for keeping you alive through consistent air supply.

The vagus nerve handles the digestive process as it is attached to the entire gastrointestinal tract from the esophagus to the colon. In other words, it controls the organs that facilitate digestion and enable the movement of bolus down to the intestines. The nutrients in the food are broken down and digested to provide the body with all the minerals and chemicals required for survival.

Its motor and sensory capabilities. Being one of the few cranial nerves that have both motor and sensory capabilities, the vagus nerve integrates its functions and combines them to ensure that the motor signals are synchronized with the sensory ones. Specifically, the motor senses enable you to make movements to balance your body or avoid danger. Notably, the motor capabilities of this nerve help it manage most body functions as it provides uniform body awareness. Surely, the senses make it easier to carry out your daily activities especially when you need to make movements in your neck and shoulders.

The sensory skills of this nerve are as necessary as the motor ones for they are the only means of passing information from the brain to other body organs. For instance, the vagus nerve enhances the bowel movement allowing the stomach emptying and release of digestive juices from the pancreas and bile. It also controls your hormones, thus regulating your reaction to the environment and situations in your life.

Easily stimulated. The vagus nerve manages to provide various functions, especially in clinical fields, for it is easily stimulated. Medical practitioners prefer stimulating the nerve to address chronic diseases and psychological conditions. In this case, the extent of the vagus nerve makes it easy to access and regulate the functioning of numerous body organs that it is attached to. There are efforts to broaden the stimulation of this nerve as it has proven to provide results that are rare in other treatments. With this form of stimulation, the patient's responsibilities are eased as they may not be needed to take regular medication.

Moreover, the exercise itself is so simple, thanks to advanced technology and the digitization of medical care. Most of the devices that stimulate the nerve are using electrical impulses that send signals to the brain and are usually controlled through a program or a magnet. On the positive side, a continued expedition of advanced stimulation of the vagus nerve could treat conditions such as cluster headache, multiple sclerosis, and rheumatoid arthritis.

The Effect Of The Vagus Nerve On Your Mind

The vagus nerve can have an effect on your memories and thought processes. It's been linked to hormone production that stimulates the fight or flight response, feelings of happiness or contentment, and the lack of these can result in an imbalance within the brain. Anxiety, depression, and other mental health issues are all affected by the vagus nerve and whether it tells the brain to produce the necessary hormones or not.

Stimulation of the nerve has proven useful in a variety of ways. Not only can a functioning vagus nerve help prevent issues like depression or anxiety, it can also be useful in building memories. If you need to remember things better or plan to study for an exam, it can actually help if you stimulate the vagus nerve. You'll remember better and it improves neuroplasticity or the ability to learn. In fact, it's even been shown to help with conditions like dementia and Alzheimer's. Some people use vagal stimulation as a method of improving their memory and learning over a longer period of time.

Can The Vagus Nerve Regenerate?

The vagus nerve manages so many parts of the body that it can be devastating when something goes wrong. If there is anything that damages the nerve, such as medication, trauma, or disease, can the body heal itself? Or are you stuck with nerve damage for the rest of your life? It really all depends on how bad the damage is.

Nerve damage is notorious for being slow to heal and the vagus nerve is no exception. However, scientists have tested the ability of the vagus nerve to regenerate in rats and the results have been surprising. Not only have vagus nerve techniques helped with the restoration of the central vagal parts, but they have also been shown to increase synaptic plasticity. This means that even when the brain suffers damage from damage done to the vagus nerve, it can be reversed, to a certain extent.

In tests done on rats, it took roughly 4.5 months to regenerate the central vagal nerve. That's good news for people, though it hasn't been fully tested in humans. However, studies have also shown that rebuilding the nerves in the gastrointestinal tract did not occur over the course of 45 weeks, or almost a year, which is how long the study lasted. It will definitely take time for nerves to grow back and regenerate, but the fact that it is actually possible could be exactly the hope we need.

While the central sections of the vagal nerve can be regenerated surprisingly quickly, it takes much longer to regrow the areas that branch out from it. It's important to note this, because you shouldn't expect instant results from the exercises and techniques given in this book.

Stimulation of the vagus nerve can help it grow and recover from damage. Again, it takes time, but if you are willing to put in the time and effort, you'll find that things gradually get better. As many people have discovered before you, this is not a trick. Vagus nerve stimulation really works and it can have an incredible impact on your life.

Even if you haven't suffered from any particular trauma or nerve damage, you can still expect some results from toning up your vagus nerve. It can only help you feel better and ensure that your body runs more efficiently. The amount of energy you'll have will increase and you will find that it is easier to live the lifestyle you want.

Chapter 2

Exercise To Activate The Vagus Nerve

Exercising isn't just good as a temporary mood boost; it's good for your entire physical health, and the benefits can be felt whether you're doing a small low-intensity exercise or lifting heavy weights multiple times a week.

Exercise is a necessary part of healing from chronic pain. You don't have to become an active bodybuilder or an athlete, but some degree of body movement is highly desirable to prevent chronic pain. Body movements release the "stuck" energy in our body and ensure a smooth flow of energy to prevent any pain.

If you do exercise more this will help with your self-esteem. Exercising will make you healthier and you will feel better about yourself. If you are worried about your health and it is making your anxiety worse, get out there and do some exercises. To really help lower anxiety, it is a good idea that each time you exercise to be sure it is for 30 minutes or more. Studies have shown that it takes about thirty minutes for your anxiety to lower when exercising.

If you don't want to exercise alone, grab a friend to do this activity with you. This will make you happy and you can have someone to talk to about the things you are anxious about. It's great to have someone who you can let all of your feelings be expressed to who can help you. Healthy exercise has some surprising implications for those with anxiety disorders and other psychological conditions including depression. The mechanisms by which exercise and mental health are related are not fully understood, but many medical experts around the world now acknowledge that exercise has a major impact on a wide range of psychological conditions. It is even now believed that exercise can be as effective at combating depression as many commonly prescribed drugs.

Short bursts of activity a few times a day are the type of exercise that experts recommend. A brisk walk lasting only ten minutes is believed to be enough to raise your emotional state for a couple of hours. For those with anxiety disorders, it can be hard to get out and about on occasion. For some, with severe conditions, it can seem impossible. Exercise, however, will really help to improve your emotional state and take your mind off anxiety.

Moderate level intensity exercise is recommended as perfect for improving your physical health and also your mental health. This includes; walking briskly, cycling, jogging or swimming. Walking and jogging should not need any investment and if you're uncomfortable alone, partner up with a friend or relative. Ideally buddy up with someone who is addressing the same issues or has a good understanding of them, for extra support.

When we exercise, the brain releases endorphins, or "feel good" chemicals that are responsible for the "high" that many people feel during and after exercise. Another benefit of exercise for those with depression is that it lends purpose and structure to each day. Outdoor exercise has been shown to be especially effective for lifting mood.

Regular exercise can help maintain a healthy weight, which can be a problem in depressed people. Exercise promotes overall wellbeing, including heart health and a toned, more muscular body. The weight-bearing aspects of exercise prevent the body from losing bone mass and decrease the risk of osteoporosis, a particular benefit for women.

People who suffer from anxiety may not be interested in exercise. When someone is overwhelmed by the stress of everyday life, working out seems less than appealing. However, research shows that exercise plays an important role in reducing anxiety symptoms.

While exercise has been clinically proven to reduce anxiety and improve mood, it can also treat a number of other health problems. Health issues can be a major anxiety trigger, and easing the symptoms of those ailments can reduce anxiety symptoms further.

In addition, exercising can help people relax. When a person exercises, their body releases hormones that produce a calming effect. Exercise also increases body temperature, which can be very relaxing. Working up a sweat is tiring, but it's a great way to calm down.

There is no getting away from the fact that physical exercise has multiple beneficial effects on our physical health. It not only improves cardiovascular health; it also helps in fat burning and weight management. Exercise has also been proven to be effective in combating stress and anxiety. When we engage in physical exercise, the body release chemicals called endorphins that have an uplifting effect on the mood and are responsible for the feel-good after effect of exercising.

Exercise is a wonderful way to stimulate your mental, and physical health. Exercise is also great for vagal tone and vagus nerve stimulation. Exercise helps to increase the growth hormones within the brain, and it also helps with the mitochondria in the brain, which of course are the powerhouses of the cells. Exercise helps reduce and reverse the cognitive decline. When you exercise, you stimulate your brain health, and also feel good. As a result, you'll directly stimulate your vagus nerve and this will be good for brain health and physical health.

If you're someone who isn't physically fit enough to do either of those, walk for about an hour a day, both during the morning and night. Get into the habit of walking; both your brain and your body will love you for it. When you are using movement in order to stimulate the vagus nerve, you are effectively teaching your vagus nerve to become more flexible. As you are able to better your vagal tone, you should start to notice that your body is more likely to be highly and fully functional, enabling you to start seeing relief.

The movements that you will discuss within this chapter will help you develop the tone that you will need to activate those parasympathetic pathways wherever and whenever you need them. As you learn to switch between the systems at will, you will find yourself happier, calmer, and likely feeling healthier as well. Remember, each of these movements will stimulate the vagus nerve in some way—they may directly stimulate it or indirectly stimulate it, but the end result is still the same: A more toned nerve that is more capable of handling anything life happens to throw its way.

Example of exercises with stimulating the vagus nerve directly.

Wave Exercises

This is a form of exercise where you will stand on a plate that moves around up and down.

Speed Walking

Speed walking, more often referred to as power walking or race walking, is a technique of walking at a rapid pace. Walking provides all of the aerobic benefits of running while steering clear of many of the injuries associated with high-impact techniques of running. The activity of walking at an increased rate then walking "normally" can help participants lose weight, tone their muscles, and also increase their mood.

Not only is speed walking valuable for the muscles and joints, but it also reinforces overall health.

Jogging

While jogging, ensure you are also deeply breathing. Don't take short breaths while doing this form of exercise as it can harm you. Ensure you are regularly breathing. Jogging will stimulate your vagus nerve and also help regulate your breathing. If you want to turn it up a notch, you can also incorporate sprinting or running rather than lightly jogging. This is a high intensity exercise.

Yoga And Meditation

Yoga and meditation are great mental and physical exercises to incorporate into your routine. These two forms of exercise are excellent ways to promote stimulation and a healthy vagus nerve. Your vagus will be stimulated and it will help promote deep breathing, increased focus, and control. Yoga can be defined as a practice based on harmonizing the mind, body, and soul. By practicing Yoga every day, you will not only explore your true self or your inner self, but also develop the feeling that you are one with nature and environment. Yoga aids the overall wellbeing of the body and focuses mainly on developing relationship with the natural world around us.

Pain is not just influenced by physical injury or illness, it is also greatly affected by our thoughts, anxiety, trauma, stress and emotions. Stress and pain are closely interrelated - you may experience pain when stressed and stress can also increase the intensity of the pain. When there is increased stress, your breathing becomes heavier, erratic and ragged. Your mood is also altered along with some tension and tightening of the muscles. These symptoms of chronic pain can even increase the toxins in the body and decrease oxygen levels.

Yoga addresses these problems effectively, as it involves the techniques of deep breathing and meditation, which helps in the absorption of much-needed oxygen and also in the relaxation of mind and body. These breathing techniques ensure that the muscles of the lungs, diaphragm, back, and abdomen are fully utilized. Stress and anxiety levels will also be reduced gradually.

Yoga, or simple stretching, are simple practices that should be applied to everyday life to reduce the tension of stress and keep the muscles in proper working order. There are specific stretches that can focus on problem areas such as the neck or lower back. These stretches can be assigned from a personal trainer, massage therapist, or physiotherapist. Yoga can be enjoyed at home or in a studio with several other participants. The focus in yoga is on breath control, meditation, stretching, and balance. Not all forms of yoga are spiritual with chants and mantras, if you don't feel comfortable with that form of practice.

Exercise in general is good for chronic pain, but specific exercises, especially certain yoga positions, help to decrease some types of pain, like shoulder or neck pain.

Additionally, the relaxation techniques you will learn, can teach you how to manage the different types of chronic pain more effectively.

Yoga itself is incredibly effective in helping you relax and activate your parasympathetic nervous system. When you are using this, you are combining yoga, breathing, and mindfulness to relax and meditate for a moment, allowing you to clear your mind while also activating that parasympathetic response that stimulates the vagus nerve.

One such pose you can use to do so is child's pose—this will involve you making sure your knees are spread as widely as possible on the floor while you sink your stomach down to the floor, between the thighs. Your feet should be flat on the ground, toes pointing behind you and tucked underneath your bottom. Your forehead will touch the floor and you will stretch your arms out as far as possible.

Within this pose, you will be stretching out all of the important nerves that are directly involved in the vagus nerve and its stimulation, allowing you to activate it, and you will also find that your stretching is comfortable and relaxing as well. Doing so enables you to start to activate those nerves and see the benefits.

When you sink into this position, remain for as long as you are comfortable—some people will enjoy it far longer than others. The important part here is to stretch gently to help yourself feel better. It is not designed to hurt. All that matters is you are stretching out within a similar pose in order to see the benefits. If you are not yet flexible enough or uncomfortable, modify the pose in any way that can help you reach that more comfortable position.

Jumping

Jumping around may make you look silly, but is a great form of exercise to try to stimulate your vagus nerve. This helps to stimulate the body while moving around. It will get your heart rate pumping and increase blood flow, promoting your body with the circulation it needs.

Weight Training

While you may not be able to deadlift 300 pounds right off the bat, start off with small weights. Start off by lifting 10 pounds, then slowly increase the weight as you get used to it. It can help with coordination, blood flow, breathing, and make you more aware of your body and movements. Be careful that you don't overexert yourself while weight training.

Aerobics

Aerobics are a great way to promote proper breathing techniques. Any fitness centre you visit will offer aerobics classes. There are many to choose from. For example, yoga, cycling, weight training, water aerobics, etc. All of these are great for vagus nerve stimulation.

Swimming

Swimming is yet again another great exercise for vagus nerve stimulation. It requires you to control your breathing as you propel your body through water. It also provides movement to your body which will encourage blood flow.

Dancing

Another great form of exercise is dancing. Look into dancing classes around your area. If there are any, consider taking a beginner class. This can be for any form of dance; just something to get your body moving and blood flow going. Similar to dance classes are zumba classes. These are interactive, fun, and active. These classes incorporate exercise and dance in one class. Any type of class that requires some form of movement, and not necessarily vigorous movement, are what will help you stay in shape, and stimulate your vagus nerve for a healthy body and living.

By dancing more, you're stimulating the body, and later the vagus nerve, which will help with improving your vagal tone. Plus, obesity, diabetes, and the like can be controlled with proper diet and exercise, which in turn will increase vagal tone.

Stretching

Stretching is something everyone should do on a regular basis, and those with chronic back pain will benefit most from stretching the soft the muscles, ligaments, and tendons in and around the spine.

It is a fact that when motion is limited the back becomes stiff, which can result in more pain. Those who suffer from chronic back pain need to stretch regularly and perform appropriate stretching movements to benefit from the sustained and long-term relief from the increased motion.

Chapter 3

How Vagus Nerve Helps Reduce Inflammation

Inflammation is not inherently a bad thing—it is a defense mechanism that the body employs to protect and heal the body. It is, essentially, a sign that your body is fighting off some sort of foreign body. This may be bacteria, or it could be a virus, or even something that has fallen out of place. Despite being a normal response by the immune system, it can also cause a myriad of issues as well, if allowed to get out of hand. It can cause pain, stiffness, and even struggles to function if the immune system goes overboard.

Your body can fight the antibodies that come in to interfere with normal functioning. The process of your body fighting these infections, injuries that want to harm you is called inflammation. Your body produces chemicals to trigger something that comes in to destroy your cells. These chemicals released cause a response from your system. This involves a high rate of the flow of blood as well as the proteins and antibodies released in the affected area. This happens instantly or can take a little more time if the inflammation was serious. On the other hand, chronic inflammation comes through when the response does not work, leaving your body numb and anxious. This chronic inflammation has long term effects if left and may hurt your parts such as the tissues. Research shows that chronic inflammation could also trigger conditions such as asthma conditions as well as cancer.

Inflammation is just one step in the process of healing. When your body is attacked by external forces, such as toxins, injuries, and infections that enter the body through openings or damages to the skin, then inflammation is a way for the body to fight against those forces. The body activates it when something damages or attacks your cells. It begins the process of inflammation by first releasing chemicals that encourage the immune system to respond.

So far, so good. Your body is only using its natural defense mechanisms to heal you. However, things take a turn for the worst when the immune response lingers for a long time. When it does, the body is forced to stay in a constant state of alertness. This adds extra stress on the body.

Acute Versus Chronic Inflammation: The Signs

When your body is going through the acute inflammation process, then you will notice symptoms such as swelling, redness, and pain in the area of damage. These symptoms are nothing you should be panicked about; they are part of the natural process of healing.

On the other hand, chronic inflammation has some serious symptoms. Here are some: chest pain, fatigue, mouth sores, abdominal pain, fever, rashes. And no, that is not the worst part about chronic inflammation. The worst part is that the aforementioned symptoms can last for several months or years. Imagine going through abdominal pain for years.

The Cause Of Chronic Inflammation

There are several causes of chronic inflammation. The most obvious ones are listed below:

- An acute inflammation response takes place and it goes untreated. For example, when you do not deal with an injury or infection, leaving it there to fester or worsen.

- Acute inflammation could be caused by an autoimmune response. This is a response that occurs when your body turns in on itself. In such cases, the immune system mistakes healthy tissues and cells as invaders and decides to attack them.
- You could also encourage chronic inflammation when your skin or a wound is exposed to irritants, such as pollution or industrial chemicals, for a long time. Eventually, your body does not get to rest because it is busy dealing with external forces constantly.

Now those are the obvious causes because you can see them develop on your body. Take the situation where your body is attacked by chemical substances. You can see the effects of it on the wound or injury. But not all causes are obvious. You might encourage chronic inflammation due to the below: chronic stress, obesity, smoking, alcohol In other words, you might not even be aware of the fact that you are causing chronic inflammation.

How Chronic Inflammation Affects Our Body

Think again about or look back at the list of symptoms of chronic inflammation. Those symptoms only touch the tip of the symptom iceberg. The real problems occur as the inflammation worsens because when it does, it targets healthy organs, tissues, and cells. It does not stop there. Over time, as your organs, tissues, and cells continue to suffer, they lead to damage to your DNA, scarring within your body, and death of tissues. What you are left with are conditions that change your life completely. Conditions such as the below: asthma, type 2 diabetes, cancer, obesity, heart disease, various neurodegenerative diseases, including Alzheimer's.

Symptoms Of Chronic Inflammation

You will be able to note when the symptoms of acute inflammation occur. This is because there are signs of foreseen symptoms such as swelling, pain, or redness. However, you should be keen because you could easily overlook them. The following are the common symptoms of chronic inflammation:

- You could feel tired of nothing much done
- You will experience mouth sores
- You may suffer from a fever
- You may have rashes all over your body
- You may feel some pain in the abdomen
- You may suffer from chest pain

Inflammation Disorders

There are other disorders that are directly related to inflammation as well, and there are also other forms of arthritis that are not necessarily associated with inflammation, so keep that in mind.

The three forms of arthritis that do relate to inflammation, however, can be incredibly painful. The first one is rheumatoid arthritis, Secondly, we have Psoriatic arthritis which is specific to people who are already suffering from psoriasis—which is a type of skin condition that results in skin that appears red, patchy, and with greyish-silver scales developing atop them. Those who suffer from psoriasis sometimes also develop psoriatic arthritis, in which your immune system attacks itself. It most often results in the swelling of fingers and toes, feeling pain within your feet, particularly where connective tissue meets bone, and pain in the lower back. This particular kind of arthritis can do serious damage to the joints, largely because the immune system is effectively targeting the joint that is healthy—despite the absence of a threat or danger, the area is attacked due to the inflammation.

Gouty arthritis, sometimes just known as gout, is a type of arthritis that is the result of uric acid levels being too high. Essentially, the uric acid solidifies within the joints, and the solid crystals of uric acid tend to form into sharp points, which then can hurt the joint. As the joint becomes hurt, then, it develops the common symptoms of arthritis as a result.

How Does Chronic Inflammation Affect Your Body?

When one is experiencing chronic inflammation, there are healthy cells that can be destroyed in your body. This includes death in tissues; healthy cells will damage, and also other parts of the body. The inflammation can further cause internal damage. A study by the medical sector further researched to see whether these effects could link to any other conditions. The study proved that several diseases were linked such as; cancer, heart disease, arthritis, diabetes, being obese, and asthma. In controlling chronic inflammation, what you eat will play both an objective and a subjective role. Foods to be consumed include a range of foods have non-inflammatory effects. Which include foods that are high in antioxidants and polyphenols, including sunflower oil green vegetables, like spinach and kale berries, fatty fish, like tuna, tuna, and salmon nuts, particularly strawberries, strawberries, and grapes.

Now we have much information about the chronic inflammation in our bodies. The next step is to take note of the treatment. You need to be aware that the reduction of inflammation starts by working on the vagus nerve.

How Is The Vagus Nerve Is Involved In Treating Chronic Inflammation?

Since the vagus nerve is the primary source for the body and brain to communicate, allowing for feedback in both directions, it is primarily responsible for identifying when there is inflammation within the body. When it is able to find that inflammation, largely through detecting cytokines, the brain finds out about that inflammation and can then make sure that the proper amount of anti-inflammatory hormones are released. This means that the inflammation is properly regulated—it is not too strong, nor is it to underwhelming.

This proper response leads to people with entirely normal, functioning inflammation levels when it is necessary. For example, when you are injured or you get a minor infection, that inflammation is necessary. The body regulates itself. However, for some people, this inflammation response can be largely suppressed, leading to immunodeficiency. Those whose response is too strong, on the other hand, can find themselves struggling with highly responsive inflammatory responses that attack themselves.

Let's say that your body has now encountered a threat in the environment. Your brain perceives said threat and sends signals to various parts of the body, activating the fight-or-flight response. Despite the state of stress you are in after your body feels the effects of working too hard, it is necessary for you to deal with the situation. Now suppose that you realize that the threat in the environment is no cause for being alert. Biologically, your body is supposed to respond to the stress, realize that the threat has passed and then calm down immediately. The brain created the fight-or-flight instincts. But it is the vagus nerve that plays the primary role in activating the parasympathetic relaxation response. It is simply the vagus nerve's way of saying, "Stop! No need to be alarmed. The threat has passed." And to do this, the vagus nerve stimulates the release of acetylcholine, a neurotransmitter that is the body's equivalent of "hitting the brakes" on the inflammation response, which also gets activated when you enter fight-or-flight.

With that, your body begins to relax. Your breathing starts slowing down. Your heartbeat, which was thumping like a drum solo in a rock concert, starts to return back to a calm rhythm.

The vagus nerve releases acetylcholine for the main purpose of stopping the inflammation process, whether it is caused by your fight-or-flight response or not. In other words, when your body is healing and if it reaches a point when injury or damage does not pose a threat, then acetylcholine stops the inflammation process.

The strength of the vagus nerve's response–or in other words, how well it can stop the inflammatory process–is called the vagus tone. When the vagus tone is low, your inflammation becomes chronic because the system responsible for telling your body to calm down does not have enough power to do so. It went from being the boss of your body's organization to a mid-level employee.

With a high vagus tone, you make sure to manage the levels of inflammation in the body.

Chapter 4

How Vagus Nerve Helps Reduce Anxiety

Stress is a normal experience that we face frequently throughout the day. Most often we deal with stressful situations without even thinking about it. We may be stressed about a new job, giving a presentation, or about your children starting their first day of school. While it is a completely normal and healthy experience, stress can lead to many mental and health disorders when we become overwhelmed or are unable to bounce out of the stressful situation.

You are waiting for an important meeting to start. The materials for the meeting are with you. Soon enough, you are tapping your feet to an unknown rhythm in your head, hoping that the meeting starts soon. No amount of telling your mind that you are overreacting is enough—you still feel like there is some sort of threat lurking around the corner.

If that sounds familiar, it is entirely possible that you could be suffering from anxiety. This means that your body is constantly feeling as though there is some imminent threat lurking around the corner, no matter how irrational it may be.

While anxiety on its own is sometimes normal, healthy, and totally expected, such as if you are going to your first day at a new job, or if you have a job interview, it is important to understand that if your anxiety has become such a constant in your life that you are always struggling, always suffering, and always attempting to get out from underneath that stress, it could be a problem in your life.

When you are anxious, your fear drive is on auto-pilot. You may feel a sense of dread deep within yourself that you cannot explain or regulate. You may feel like you have no way to stop those feelings of fear and dread, and oftentimes, it can be incredibly difficult to do so if you are not armed and prepared. It can manifest as phobias, as obsessions and compulsions, or as panic attacks. Other times, it can manifest as just a deep-seated feeling of dread and terror. Nevertheless, it is important to recognize just how that anxiety can impact your life.

Types Of Anxiety Disorders

Panic Disorder

Panic disorder can strike individuals at any time without warning or logical explanation. These types of stress disorders create an intense feeling of fear because the individuals never know when a panic attack with occur. These attacks can occur in highly stressful situations such as at the office when having to meet with your boss or during typical daily routines like making a pot of coffee.

Social Anxiety Disorders

Social anxiety disorders are anxiety disorders associated with the fear of being judged by others. This type of anxiety disorder can make it impossible for individuals to make connections with others, keep a job, or even leave their house. Social anxiety disorder can cause individuals to become obsessive about the way they look, dress, act, and their lifestyle. Individuals can often feel themselves trapped by the need to please everyone and to make everyone like them. They will often ruminate or think and replay social interactions in their heads negatively, finding all the things they should have done differently.

Obsessive-Compulsive Disorder

Obsessive-compulsive disorder tends to present repetitive actions that are encouraged by illogical thoughts. Individuals can find themselves having to repeat patterns until done correctly, repeating actions a specific number of times, or needing to have things strategically placed in specific locations. Obsessive-compulsive disorder can hinder an individual's way of life as it can lead to feeling embarrassed or ashamed because of their obsessive behaviors. Individuals struggle to make connections with others because they never feel understood. Most individuals with obsessive-compulsive disorder struggle to make sense of why they feel the need to perform the repetitive behavior themselves and simply stopping can trigger serious panic attacks that leave them immobile.

Illness Anxiety Disorder

Illness anxiety disorders refer to those that can arise from somatic disorders. With this type of anxiety disorder, individuals become obsessively concerned about their health. Many individuals with illness anxiety disorder are diagnosed with hypochondria. Hypochondria can cause individuals to believe intensely that they have a serious health condition that they then actually begin to manifest the symptoms of that condition.

Phobias

Phobias can revolve around objects, activities, people, animals, and/or situations, and they can cause individuals to become temporarily paralyzed when confronted with the phobia. Phobias can cause an irrational fear response in the body, which can be a minor response or debilitating response. Often individuals can avoid their phobias and go about their daily routine without it affecting them; other individuals are unable to avoid these situations. Those with a fear of small spaces, wide space, heights, or common animals like dogs may have more difficulty living their lives fully.

Symptoms Of Anxiety Disorders

Anxiety symptoms can vary greatly from person to person. Each person will feel anxiety in a different way from those around them. This means that some people will report having several different symptoms of anxiety, while others will report having none. There are no specific symptoms or presentation of symptoms that must be present in order to diagnose—in order to get a diagnosis, rather, you must show that you have any number of anxiety symptoms that are severe enough that they are directly impacting your life for the worse. While each type of anxiety disorder can impact individuals differently, many, despite their specific type of anxiety, will often experience some common symptoms. These symptoms can include:

- Rapid heart rate
- Increasing in breathing
- Feeling restless
- Inability to concentrate
- Unable to sleep.

Anxiety attacks are also regularly experienced by most individuals. Anxiety attack can happen suddenly and cause:

- Fainting
- Dizziness
- Difficulty breathing
- Dry mouth
- Increase in sweating
- Hot flashes
- Excessive worry

- Feeling amped up or restless
- Distress
- Fear
- Numbing or tingling sensation throughout the body.

Stress And The Nervous System

It takes charge of your body's mechanisms to make sure you are prepared to deal with the stressful situation, as we had seen earlier where increased heart rate, improved focus, and other such reactions are enabled to help you.

But simply talking about the autonomic nervous system is like telling everyone that an airplane flies in the sky.

When you experience stress, then your automatic reaction is to try and either deal with the stress itself or the situation that causes it. For some people, working with stress is not as bad as it is for others. They have a high threshold. But when people cannot deal with stress for a prolonged period of time, then it can lead to inflammation.

Unfortunately, at this point, the extent of knowledge that the scientific and medical communities have about the way stress causes inflammation breaks down. There is no accurate information that can explain just why stress can contribute to inflammation. But the conclusion is that it does.

In one corner, we have stress and its choice of weapon, inflammation. In the other corner, we have the vagus nerve–with a little help from the ANS–and its choice of weapons, all the good chemicals. The fight is not going to be easy. Any side can take the upper hand. It all depends on one factor—you.

Your body is filled with incredible defense mechanisms. However, it cannot do everything on its own. Remember how we talked about giving your body the right fuel? That is important because it not only powers various processes, but also takes care of the warriors of our bodies, the immune system. But along with the immune system, we also have to take care of the warrior of our nervous system.

How Is The Vagus Nerve Is Involved In Treating Anxiety Disorders?

When under stress or feeling anxious, it is likely that breathing becomes shallow, short, and challenging. Stress impairs the regulation of the heart rate; the vagus nerve is often shut off because the sympathetic system becomes activated, and thus, a spiral of overwhelm and fear overtake behaviors and emotional expression.

When a situation becomes too overwhelming, the dorsal vagus nerve, or the primitive branch, steps in to cause a shut down. When this occurs, all systems are halted. Even when the dangers pass and you bounce out of the freeze and shut down response, you still remain on high alert or in fight or flight response. The vagus nerve remains inactive. Only when the individual feels safe and secure will the nerve be reactivated.

In this time of shut down and fight or flight response, the heart rate is elevated, breathing becomes irregular, and muscles remain tense.

A lack of the vagus nerve activating, then, allows for the sympathetic nervous system to run amok, allowed to rule the body altogether. It creates an increase in stress hormones, which then triggers inflammation, which can impact the brain.

Beyond that, however, the longer the sympathetic nervous system is allowed to rule, the more stressed and anxious the body becomes, creating higher levels of cortisol and glutamate, both of which stress out the body even further. This means that you are left feeling miserable.

Exercises To Activate The Vagus Nerve To Reduce Anxiety And Stress

Because it is inevitable then you will encounter some form of stress, vagal nerve stimulation multiple times a day can allow you to easily move on from it. By stimulating the vagus nerve when facing a stressful situation, you can disrupt the sympathetic systems fight or flight response. This, in turn, can allow you to return to a calmer and peaceful state. Stimulating the vagus can allow you time to properly assess the situation, which can lead to better choices being made. The best way to stimulate the vagus nerve when stressed is through deep breathing exercises and cold temperatures.

Deep Breathing

Deep breathing is done by inhaling, then performing a long exhale. The inhale slightly increases the heart rate while the long exhale will decrease the heart rate. This results in a lower overall heart rate that also lowers blood pressure and this is a highly effective way to stimulate the vagus nerves.

When you practice deep breathing when facing a stressful situation, you allow yourself to take control of your reactions and thoughts. Taking a minute to simply breathe in and out deeply triggers a calming response. This, in turn, allows you to think more clearly and communicate effectively.

Diving Reflex

You can instantly halt the sympathetic nerves and activate the vagus nerve by performing what is called the diving reflex. This can be done by splashing cold water on the face, holding an ice pack or ice cubes against the face, or drinking cold water and holding it in your mouth. As you apply the cold sensation, you want to hold your breath in temporarily. Doing this causes your blood pressure to lower and your heart rate to slow down. Your body should instantly feel more relaxed and calm as the anxiety subsides.

Chapter 5

How Vagus Nerve Helps Reduce Depression

Along with anxiety, another commonly occurring mental health issue is depression. When you feel depressed, you may struggle with your own thoughts. Many people around the world struggle with depression, with an estimated 300 million people suffering. It is nearly as common as anxiety, and of those people, nearly 50% of them also get diagnosed with an anxiety disorder as well, leading to a double hit of mental health issues all at one time, causing serious struggle for them. At any given point, roughly 15% of the adult population will go through some sort of depressive episode during their life. You may have a few days where you feel more down and blue than others but this isn't necessarily depression even if that is how you describe what you are feeling to others. Depression is much more complex and debilitating than feeling sad. This is a condition that invokes feelings of sadness and hopelessness. It is a mood disorder that can alter your mood, behavior, and physical health. Depression can cause individuals to lose interest in many areas of their lives and result in significant struggles to perform even the simplest of tasks. Everything feels like a burden and inconvenience; these feelings are a reflection not just of how the individual views their surrounding but also how they view themselves.

Depression Symptoms

Depression, despite the myriad of symptoms that it brings about with it, is largely treatable. You can get relief from these symptoms, whether through medication, learning to regulate your vagus nerve in hopes of alleviating symptoms, learning to manage through therapy, or any other treatment method that is discussed between you and a doctor. Please remember—if you ever feel as though you are thinking about harming yourself, you should treat this as a medical emergency and you should seek out emergency treatment immediately.

- Low mood: When you are depressed, you almost always struggle to function effectively. Your mood fails to regulate and you feel down the vast majority of the time. Keep in mind that those are depressed may not always show signs of depression 100% of the time—they may be depressed some of the time but seem fine the rest of the time. It is entirely dependent on the individual that is being considered at that moment in time.
- Change in appetite: You may find yourself endlessly hungry or entirely uninterested in eating altogether thanks to your depression.
- Sleep disturbances: As with eating, you may find yourself sleeping constantly or not at all. You may find yourself suffering from extreme insomnia or feeling the urge to sleep constantly without ever feeling rested.
- Irritated and agitated: You fail to regulate your mood regularly due to the fact that you are constantly depressed and feeling negative. Those negative feelings very quickly give way to irritation when things do not go your way.
- Fatigued: No matter how much sleep you may get, you always feel exhausted and fatigued. Sometimes, even getting out of bed can seem like too much effort.

- Struggling to concentrate: You frequently struggle to concentrate, feeling like your mind is sluggish and struggling to function.
- Lack of interest: Everything that used to bring you enjoyment and pleasure now seems bland and dull in comparison. You find little to no pleasure in anything that you could possibly do.
- Feelings of guilt and worthlessness: You may feel as though you are worthless or guilty of something that you did not do in the first place, despite the fact that you do not have anything to feel guilty for. Especially if you are struggling to function on a daily basis, you may feel like you are letting your friends and family down.
- Fixation on death or suicide: You may self-harm, or you may strongly consider suicide, and may even spend time coming up with plans to make those thoughts a reality, even if that is not something you feel like you would ever go through with. Sometimes, the hopelessness can just seem too overwhelming.

Causes Of Depression

Hereditary elements are significant much of the time of depression. Depression appears to run in families, and about 30% of the inclination for depression is because of hereditary impacts.

Stressful life occasions influence the beginning or backslide of depression. Promoting and facilitating strife, malice, or resentment can badly have a grave effect on our success and mental health, as also, different issues and ecological stressors, for example, budgetary challenges, retirement, joblessness, labor, forlornness, or loss of a person or thing significant. In helpless individuals, these undesirable life occasions might be sufficient to cause or intensify a burdensome ailment.

An individual's characteristics are peculiar points that determines the person's wellbeing. At a particular time in life when they lack encouragement, they will for the most part, have an exceptionally negative perspective on themselves and the world. They don't acknowledge beneficial things, and awful things appear to be overpowering. A few people tend to see things this way in any event, when they are not discouraged. As such, they may have a burdensome character style.

Just as with any emotion, feeling sad is a healthy part of keeping your mind-body connection strong. Sadness can lead to feelings of gratitude for the happier moments. Sadness can also serve as a reminder to stay present at the moment. This emotion can bring on tears, regret, guilt, or shame. While it is healthy to go through short periods of sadness, it isn't an emotion you want to get stuck on. When you begin to feel sadness more often than feeling happy, you might find yourself falling into depression.

How Is The Vagus Nerve Is Involved In Treating Depression?

A lack of serotonin is evident in many individuals with depression. Serotonin is a hormone that is primarily produced in the digestive tract. When released, it plays a role in regulating sleep cycles, suppressing appetite, and promoting feelings of well-being and happiness. When the parasympathetic system is active, the vagus nerve can effectively send these signals; when the sympathetic system is in command, the vagus nerve has a difficult time bypassing the signals sent out by the sympathetic nervous system, which results in a reduction of serotonin being produced.

Despite the fact that most forms of depression can be treated with less invasive methods, the fact that vagus nerve stimulation can treat depression implies that there is some involvement there. While it is not entirely known why stimulating the vagus nerve will trigger an improvement in depression, especially treatment resistant depression that has been difficult to treat in the first place, it has been found to be effective.

Just as with anything, moderation is key—some stress is good, and can even be motivational, but when the sympathetic nervous system is free to rule the mind, inflammation begins to occur.

That inflammation in particular could potentially be related to depression. The inflammation lessens serotonin levels within the brain, which then leads to mood regulation problems.

The implication, then, is that the lack of stimulation from the vagus nerve allows the sympathetic nervous system to run rampant. That causes an inflammatory response within the body, which then also creates the response in which the body struggles to produce enough serotonin. That lack of serotonin, then, is linked to the depressive symptoms.

Exercises To Stimulate The Vagus Nerve To Combat Depression Symptoms

Vagus nerve stimulation can help those with treatment-resistant depression find the relief they are desperate for and can also give those on multiple medications for depression an effective alternative. Using a vagus nerve stimulator in addition to traditional therapy has been shown to significantly reduce depressive symptoms in patients (Sigrid, 2018). Aside from the vagus nerve stimulator, Sudarshan Kriya Yoga and Loving Kindness Meditation have been two effective techniques that tone and activate the vagus nerve and can be used as a form of a natural antidepressant.

Sudarshan Kriya Yoga

Yoga focuses on strengthening the mind-body connection. Kriya yoga is a focused breathing type of yoga that aims to balance the body's natural energy levels. While performing this type of yoga, you will alternate between fast and slow breaths, which stimulates the vagus nerve and allows you to turn the parasympathetic nervous system on, passing into the social engagement phase of calm and security. This yoga sequence involves these basic steps:

Bhastrika Pranayama

- Remain in a seated crossed leg position. Keep the right hand resting on the right knee.
- Inhale through the nose so you can fill your stomach and lungs with air.
- Strongly exhale through the nose in short shallow breaths. As you exhale, you want to use the left hand on the abdomen to help push the air out by rhythmically pushing on the abdomen.
- Continue the rhythmic breathing and abdomen pushing for a full 30 seconds. Then allow yourself to take a few relaxed natural breaths.
- Take another deep inhale through the nose and repeat the process for five minutes.

Sudarshan Kriya

- Remain in the same seated position with the palms facing up.
- Balance the breath, where you inhale and exhale for the same length of time at least five times.
- On the next inhale sequence, you want to keep your inhales and exhales the same length but double the time it takes to perform them. For example, if your regular sequence of breathing is four seconds of inhaling and four seconds of exhaling, you want to take eight seconds to inhale and eight seconds to exhale. Repeat this inhale, exhale sequence five times.
- Finally, you want to keep the length of the inhale longer, at twice the normal speed, but shorten the exhale. If you are inhaling for eight seconds, you exhale will last for only four seconds. Repeat this breathing sequence five times. Then return to your normal breathing pattern.

Loving Kindness Meditation

The Loving Kindness Meditation is a specific type of meditation that focuses on bringing love and kindness to yourself and others. It is a type of mediation that you can build on as you become more comfortable. When you first perform the Loving Kindness Meditation, you will focus most of your energy on yourself; over time you can extend this focus to other people or things in your life. Loving Kindness Meditation works to activate the vagus nerve by intentionally focusing your thoughts on feelings of love, compassion, and kindness. When the vagus nerve is activated in this way, it triggers the relaxation response in the body and serotonin is released.

- Once your breathing is calm and your body is relaxed, bring your focus to yourself. Visualize yourself feeling both physically and emotionally at peace. Imagine what it would feel like to experience a perfect type of love. Then give thanks to yourself, give thanks for all the things you are capable of, and specifically identify a few qualities about yourself that make you uniquely you. Give thanks to those qualities and allow yourself to feel at peace with who you are, just the way you are at this moment.
- As you are visualizing this inner peace and surrounding yourself with love, also imagine that with each inhale, you bring in more love and peace and with each exhale you are releasing tension.
- Add loving phrases or affirmation about yourself
- Allow yourself to feel submerged in the feelings of peace and love as you continue to inhale and exhale. If you notice your thoughts have wandered off, bring the focus back to visualizing how you would experience this kind of love. Continue to keep this focus on yourself for the remainder of the mediation session.
- When you are done meditating, slowly open the eyes. Remind yourself of how the loving kindness visualization brought you

inner peace and feelings of security and calm. When you go about your day, remember to recall upon those feelings to help you maintain a level of happy feelings by taking in a few deep inhales and exhales.

- As you become more confident and add more time to your session, you can begin to bring this loving kindness to those you care about in your life. You can do this after step six. Here you would bring a specific person into your visualization, and just as you imagined yourself feeling inner peace and love, you will now imagine this other person receiving these types of positive feelings.
- Once you have sent loving kindness to one person, try again with another and continue the process until you have completed your session.

Chapter 6

How Vagus Nerve Helps Control Your Anger

Allowing yourself to consciously express the anger you feel is very healthy, not only emotionally, but also physically. Repressed anger makes people sick. It causes a person to turn their anger toward themselves. This pent-up anger usually leads to people feeling drained and depressed. The problem is that we haven't been really taught how to express our emotions in a healthy manner, which is why we often end up stuffing all our feelings inside, especially anger.

On the contrary, we have been taught to avoid anger and other feelings related to it. But if you come to think of it, our emotions, including anger, are there for a reason. Instead of going against your anger when you're feeling like you want to explode, decide to go with the flow. But then again, make sure you know how to safely express your anger, so that you avoid hurting other people and avoid hurting yourself.

Anger is an extremely potent emotion that can originate from any multitude of feelings such as disappointment, sadness, hurt, resentment, etc. It's a standard emotion that everyone has felt and that everyone feels differently, whether they are mildly annoyed or enraged. It's natural to feel anger no matter what the strength of that anger is. Anger can range from minor irritation to steady frustration, to blind rage. Any amount of anger a person feels should be validated, just as a person's depression, anxiety, happiness, etc. should be. Anger is not just an emotional response, but it is also a physical response within the body. When you begin to feel angry, your body produces extra adrenaline and cortisol, which are "stress hormones." This causes your blood to travel faster to the muscles in your arms and legs in order to allow your body to physically react fast enough to avoid the threat that it recognizes your anger as. This causes less blood in your brain, causing the thought process to become "cloudy." So, while you are feeling your anger mentally, the rest of your body is feeling it too.

Anger can be caused by multiple things internally or externally. Things like negative thought patterns are an internal stimulus that can cause anger, while an external stimulus could be something happening due to another person that is outside of your control. Indeed, anger can essentially be referred to as a moral emotion due to it coming forward in times of injustice against oneself or others. Though justified in those types of situations, it can cause a person to go too far with their defense when they are not under control. Without techniques or a plan to control yourself when you are feeling angry, your anger can become a big problem.

Using anger as a coping mechanism is not a healthy way to approach any sort of problem and can lead to it becoming too much to handle. When anger goes uncontrolled it can have a harmful effect on the person feeling it, in addition to the other people that interact with them. The effect it has on mental health can lead to more problematic issues like strained romantic or familial relationships, strained friendships, poor work performance, poor academic performance, etc. In some extremes, it can even lead to more serious problems or actions such as physical abuse, emotional abuse, substance abuse, and other criminal activity due to the lack of impulse control and aggression that can result from untreated anger problems. Aggression is the feeling of actually wanting to cause harm to someone physically or mentally, so when a person's anger is building up within them, they may start to act out aggressively toward others and hurt someone else or themselves. That is the main reason that anger needs to be under control, to prevent anyone from being hurt.

When it goes unmanaged, it focuses more on the emotional moment and the perceived problem rather than finding a solution. This is another reason why managing it is important, because you may feel less stressed and have better problem-solving skills in the long run. Anger is also connected with the concept of the instincts fight, flight, and freeze. Anger is one of the driving forces behind the "fight" instinct, meaning that anger allows your brain and body to choose fighting as an option when it is necessary in times of self-preservation. This is an important reason that anger should be regulated within everyone so that their brains and bodies stay alert and are able to be stimulated when necessary, rather than in times that you are lacking control of yourself.

Chronic, unmanaged anger has been linked to many different health complications;

- Digestive issues
- High blood pressure
- Skin problems
- Joint pain
- Insomnia
- Dizziness/lightheadedness
- Ulcers
- Strokes
- Hormonal imbalances
- Chronic headaches
- An increase in anxiety levels
- Depression

- Hypertension
- Eczema and other skin conditions
- Heart attack

When all of these different physical reactions are happening at a frequent rate, it can possibly lead to permanent physical problems when left non-maintained. When someone is having some, or even all, of these physical and mental ailments due to anger, that means it has started to dominate their life and needs to be addressed.

While learning to cope with your anger can help many of these conditions to disappear, the long-term damage may already be done in some cases and it can take you much longer to heal. Looking at the last condition, how many people actually realize that frequent bouts of anger can exponentially raise their risks of a heart attack?

How Is The Vagus Nerve Is Involved In Dealing With Anger?

The vagus nerve is responsible for managing the relaxed state in which people are able to rest. However, just as with anger, when the vagus nerve is unable to trigger the parasympathetic nervous system to rule the body, the sympathetic nervous system is allowed to reign supreme over the body, wreaking its havoc as it continues for too long. The vagus nerve, of course, is going to be sending impulses back to your brain to fill it in with how the body is feeling, due to its afferent status. The longer this anger goes on as well, the less likely it is that the parasympathetic nervous system will kick into play in the first place, meaning that you will be less likely to be able to defeat that anger at any given point in time. Unless you are able to kick-start your vagus nerve back in gear to get it moving, you are going to struggle.

Exercises To Stimulate The Vagus Nerve To Combat Anger Symptoms

A common technique used in managing anger is taking slow and deep breaths. The mechanism behind this is that deep breathing activates the vagus nerve and enables it to restore the body to a relaxed and rested state. This is crucial when it comes to stress management. People with poor vagal activity are prone to chronic stress and depressive tendencies because their fight and flight response system are not being sufficiently kept in check by the vagus nerve.

Scream Inside Your Room

While it's still unclear what effects screaming will have on the individual, it's certain that many people believe such practice is a great way to let your emotions out. If you're going to scream, though, see to it that you do it inside your room and with your face covered as screaming may have negative effects on those who hear it.

Exercise

Anger is normally a result of frustration and anxiety and countless studies have shown that exercise relieves anxiety and depression.

Physical exercise also burns off the excess energy and releases endorphins into the blood that lift your mood, hence the term, "runners high". It reduces blood pressure, which is also a factor in anger, be it the cause or a result.

Breathing Therapy

One of the most prominent techniques in anger management is teaching ways to control your breathing in a way that assists in de-escalating anger. These deep breathing exercises can act as a momentary distraction. It's actually more than just a distraction, it's the reversal of your body's biological response to angry feelings. Controlled breathing in situations of anger sends a signal through the body to help it begin to calm after the release of adrenalin sent through the body. It also helps the body return to a balanced level of carbon dioxide and oxygen, rather than the unbalanced levels that happen when the body is feeling tension.

Massage Therapy

Massage is generally seen as a way of relaxing and "chilling out" as well as treating specific issues, such as pain, range of movement, etc.

Massage therapy can also help you to sleep better at night, which leaves you feeling more rested and able to cope with whatever the day throws at you without resorting to angry outbursts. Regular massage therapy is a good idea for anyone who struggles with anger and is prone to emotional outbursts.

Meditate To Relax Your Mind

You will eventually learn to worry only about what is important and let the small stuff get away, reliving your mind of tension, worry and anxiety. Meditation is one of the more powerful forms of holistic treatment. When you get angry or stressed out, your adrenal glands secrete cortisol – the angrier you get, the more cortisol is released and this leads to tight muscles, hypertension, racing heart and a surge of adrenaline. Meditation works by rebalancing the cortisol, giving your body a much-needed break and the ability to think more clearly.

Meditation also helps to melt away feelings of stress, anxiety and depression, all of which are causes of anger. It teaches you how to be the master of your emotions and it raises your threshold for stress, making it less likely that you will lose your temper and succumb to the dark energy of anger.

The third benefit of meditation is that it boosts the production of serotonin in your body. Serotonin is known as the "feel good" hormone and, when it is released, it produces feeling of euphoria and happiness, creating a high state of awareness and leaving you feeling much cooler and calmer.

Pray, Smile And Keep Faith

Prayer is one of the best forms of support and reassurance that can help to keep you free from anxiety. Developing a habit of praying and chanting daily can help to fill you with positive energy, help to calm the mind and instill a sense of faith that the world and all in it is taken care of by a higher power. Also, make an effort to smile more often, as it will make you feel happier and instill you with a sense of confidence and positivity.

Sing Or Dance

Singing or dancing in itself won't get rid of the anger you're feeling inside. Moreover, when you're doing creative things like dancing or singing, it's almost impossible to fix your mind on other things--your anger, for instance--since you're focused on what you're doing. Singing and dancing can help you be fully in the present and help you welcome distractions from the issues of life at the same time.

Chapter 7

Stopping Smoking And Drinking With Vagus Nerve

Smoking has a variety of effects on the body. The most important effect is that the stomach can produce even more gastric acid. Gastric acid is a key component of food digestion. If gastric acid is not high enough, food breakdown is not complete.

The main reason for gastric acid is usually to start the protein description and ready to break down certain minerals and vitamins later on intake into the gut. With far too little acidity the individual gets stomach pain through the gut from unprocessed foods and will eventually experience a lack of minerals and vitamins.

As a way for the stomach to absorb the food, it will work to get the required amount of acidity by

Therefore, if you want to stop smoking, you should clear the vagus nerve. Any kinesiologist or chiropractor can do this with a simple little procedure that only takes a few minutes. You will have less motivation to get a cigarette and today you can quit without signs of withdrawal and without nicotine gum or hypnosis.

You will also achieve a selection of good side effects with optimum stomach acidity. Typically, you get a far better digestion and better absorption of nutrients. A variety of irritable bowel syndrome (IBS) patients are multiple and their heartburn will vanish.

Due to much better digestion, the immune protection improves and you are less sensitive to human-made fibers, like Polyester, in a few allergies.

Researchers in the field of substance recovery have found that there could be some support for all people with drug dependence in a brand-new type of treatment.

How Is The Vagus Nerve Is Involved In Stopping Smoking And Drinking?

Obviously, this particular study began with a few animal tests with good results and these findings were probably capable of being used to treat human addiction.

However, the FDA has approved vagus nerve stimulation therapy as a cure for many health problems including clinical depression, epilepsy and discomfort, which means that this is not quite recent, causing concern or doubt. In fact, the proven benefits seem to have increased throughout the year.

vagus nerve stimulation therapy does not alleviate the symptoms of drug abuse, but drastically reduces the drive to find and consume those substances. Since the desire to go alongside its cravings and causes is an immense part of the problem, this is a major step towards making a meaningful change in the industry.

And exactly what does this new treatment do for people and all those who try to overcome addiction? For the research-related rodents, it has contributed to synaptic plasticity improvements between the prefrontal cortex and amygdala in laboratory cocaine-sufficient rats.

Simply put, it affects the brain so that it rewrites what interaction with drugs has now rewritten. Instead of falling victim to these dangerous pulls, which have been made available themselves by the chemical substances, this brand-new strategy replaces brand new reward behavior.

Since the vagus nerve is very long, it plays a major role in human brain functions and that is one of the factors that makes this particular treatment so useful.

Stimulating this nerve with some electric pulses helps experts to through their cravings according to the great impact of the nerve. We always try to eradicate the link between shooting and becoming a perceived reward, and this is almost exclusively why drugs are being consumed extensively.

If there is clearly no pleasing feeling of chasing, people are unlimitedly unlikely to take part in drug use, particularly if they are aware of risks and consequences at present.

Vagus Nerve Stimulation Therapy To Eliminate Drug Cravings

Addiction to any substance can make the life of a person topsy-turvy. By shelling out a lot to deceiving own family members, an individual fan of illegal substances can visit any degree. But just how does addiction force somebody to put a lot at stake and then shed all?

Cravings are a major problem that torments many people fighting drug addiction, particularly whenever they attempt to come from the addictive substance. Ironically, a lot of individuals will have properly attained long-range sobriety when cravings didn't arise with addiction. Apart from being viewed as the main hurdles in healing treatment, cravings are additionally the real cause of relapse.

A total recovery from addiction occurs just when an individual is devoid of cravings. Living a drug free life without the demand for frequent monitoring against drug cravings might be hard for a recovering person.

Drug cravings are successfully treated with vagus nerve stimulation treatment. Placed under the therapy, the individuals are trained new behaviors that change their old addictive behavior of seeking medicines.

Job of vagus nerve stimulation found addiction recovery In the Faculty of Texas at Dallas review, the scientists discovered the vagus nerve stimulation therapy helped individuals to recuperate from the maladaptive behavior of drug taking.

Vagus nerve stimulation it's essentially a medical practice whereby a device is implanted to a wire threaded across the vagus nerve that travels up from the neck on the mind and links together with the region accountable for regulating mood.

Sized as tiny as a silver dollar, the unit functions the same as a pacemaker. It mainly functions by delivering some electrical pulses with the vagus nerve that further reaches towards the human brain, therefore managing the cravings and urges.

VNS helps with "extinction learning" of drug seeking actions by lowering cravings and updating the behavior related to addiction with innovative ones. "Extinction of afraid memories and extinction of drug seeking memories depends on similar substrate in the human brain.

Although addicting things do well in temporarily relieving physical and emotional discomforts of drug abusers, they have to finally deal with the agonizing symptoms of substance abuse. Besides developing a selection of mental and physical problems, a lot of those individuals also become suicidal and self-destructive in nature.

Addiction to any substance could be life threatening. Just an extensive treatment program concerning detoxification, medicines, and psychotherapies and other experiential therapies as yoga, meditation etc. can assist a private get sober.

Additionally, a holistic healing management strategy is also crucial that you maintain the time of sobriety and control cravings.

Nevertheless, the degree to that healthcare providers can garner success in the treatment for drug addiction is determined by the medical attributes of the individuals that could differ based on the drug type being abused in addition to its duration, and quantity way of utilizing the medication (intravenous or oral).

Chapter 8

How Vagus Nerve Helps Heal From Disorders

Tinnitus Treatment

This particular problem can easily affect your ear and it is called a ringing noise, but it may also have high-pitched wails, rattling, rushing sound or a low-tone beep. The ear ringing can usually occur if it is subjected to the best sound, which destroys the cells in the inner ear, which sends audio information to human mind.

The human mind attempts to amend the missed signals, which leads to what are described as fantastic sounds. The injuries and definitely the standard practice of growing older are other factors behind the ear ringing.

American research workers studied the topic of "tinnitus rats" which are expected to lead to improvements in auditory cortex and that's the mind department that responds to the noise.

In revitalizing the vagus nerve, a large nerve passing from your head and neck into the abdominal region by using a small electrode electrically and engaging in several high-pitched tones simultaneously, these individuals are able to remove ears from the test subjects.

Remedied test subjects exhibited responses that suggested that the journal Nature described had stopped the tinnitus. Creatures that did not use the drug to produce the symptoms of tinnitus.

Electric stimulation of the vagus nerve remains ideal for chronic depression and controls intractable epileptic convulsions. Moreover, when it comes to good therapy in these days it can reduce noise in people with tinnitus.

Obesity Treatment

Though it is not commonly considered a disease, obesity is more than a superficial occurrence—it is not just about looks, but about health as well. When you are obese, you risk developing a myriad of other health issues, ranging from heart disease to cancer. Those who suffer from obesity have excess body fat, and for some people, that weight is harder to shed than for others.

Obesity has all sorts of risk factors—it could be caused due to hormones, genetics, or simply bad habits, such as eating too much without exercising. Oftentimes, those who are obese eat more than those who are of healthy sizes, and may also eat due to their own feelings as a way to sort of self-soothe.

Overweight is a major public health issue, affecting an estimated 650 million people. Hypertension, osteoarthritis, dyslipidemia, cardiovascular disease, diabetes and sleep apnea are common and serious problems with obesity.

Standard therapies include diet, perform therapy, exercise, and medications. Regardless of therapy, many patients fail to maintain a typical weight.

Picky nerve stimulation is still tried as obesity therapy with mixed results. Products used to provide the vagus nerve pulses in the stomach and just above the diaphragm, typically call for a major intrusive implantation procedure that exposes the patient to a medical hazard.

VA researchers have found that the repeated stimulation of the left vagal trunk in the cervix over long periods leads to a reliable and consistent decrease in excess weight.

Work with VNS for epilepsy has been a consistent loss of weight for more than a season, and several of the most obese persons have continued to lose weight. The weight loss was commensurate with the initial incidence of obesity.

On that basis, the study group developed a technique to reduce weight by stimulating the vagus nerve within the neck of a person. A neurostimulator is inserted in the chest under the epidermis under a minimally invasive procedure in this particular strategy.

The system delivers electrical impulses to one or both vagus nerve branches. Variables consisting of current amplitude, pulse rate, pulse width and an alternating duty cycle could be regulated.

Neurostimulation means of losing some weight without entering the abdomen or thorax Profile of good patients are all those with a BMI of more than 30

Positioning in the neck provides easy connection to the vagus nerve and only requires anesthesia in the ambulatory treatment Local stimulation is constantly, periodically or as per patient's Stimulation is performed continuously.

When it comes to obesity, the vagus nerve regulates the digestive system. This means that the individual's digestive system is going to respond to the vagus nerve. It will entirely regulate based on feedback by the vagus nerve—the nerve will determine whether your brain receives the message that you have eaten your fill or not, which then impacts how much you eat. Obesity, ultimately, is usually associated with the vagus nerve losing sensitivity for some reason—having a poorly responding vagus nerve means that the signal that tells your brain that you are full is too quiet. Effectively, then, the vagus nerve's dysfunction can, in some instances, be attributed to the obesity.

Cancer Treatment

Today, new research suggests that vagal nerve activation can also be much more likely to predict the survival of patients with chronic or metastatic breast cancer. To date, tumor cycle, genetic expression, age, inflammatory variables and organ function have driven cancer prognoses.

The relationship between yoga, the vagus nerve and the cancer cell is increasingly geared towards practices of consciousness such as meditation and yoga, which stimulate the nervous vagus function.

As greater vagus nerve activation affects the development of advanced stage cancer, the effect of cancer cell growth is likely to be moderated and life expectancy increased for those with advanced stage cancer. Future studies are clearly needed to support this proposal.

Vagus nerve pastime is known as vagal tone. Lower vagal tones are recommended to slow tumor growth, as they inhibit tumor mechanisms such as oxidative stress, agitation and increased activation of the sympathetic nervous system (SNS).

The vagus nerve also innerves major systemic organs, with most tumors, including the kidneys, intestines, colons and pancreas.

Vagal tone is measured by the assessment of arrythmia of the respiratory sinus. The rhythmic increase and decrease in heart rate which is synchronous with respiration are defined in the breathing sinus arrhythmias.

The pulse rate rises during inhalation (control of the sympathetic nervous system) and the vagal effect decreases. Nevertheless, the heart rate decreases during exhalation as the vagus effect increases (activation of the parasympathetic nervous system).

Higher levels of breathing sinus arrhythmia suggest greater vagal tone which also reflects the body's ability to react to environmental and metabolic challenges.

Tumor growth before time Patients with vagal tone are increasing medical experts ' interest in evaluating the development of tumor because it is linked to the autonomous performance of the nervous system and the innervation of several visceral organ systems.

In a single study in Belgium, 72 people with colorectal cancer and 113 individuals who received an Electrocardiogram (ECG) examination had been tested earlier in their treatment. ECG has a degree of arrythmia of the respiratory sinus.

In addition, tumor production markers such as Prostate Specific Antigen (PSA) were tested for all those with carcinoembryonic antigen and prostate cancer (CEA) in all people with colorectal cancer at the sixth follow-up month.

In persons with prostate cancer, the cancer stage varying from one to four (small tumor that has not spread to the surrounding tissue) predicts greater PSA levels at 6 months' follow-up, but only for persons with lower vagal tone (reduced HRV). Such findings remained consistent even after all care and age factors were taken into account.

Similarly, one year ago the cancer stage highly anticipated CEA rates for everyone with colorectal cancer, but only for all those with limited HRV even after management of all treatment and age causes. Increased overall vagal voice, combined with decreased tumor burden (number of cancer cells or cancer cells in the body) for all metastatic cancer patients.

This particular study is one of the first of its kind to show the possible moderator of vagal tone as measured using HRV for colorectal cancer and prostate growth. The authors suggest that the vagal tone could be of interest to all those with advanced phase cancer as a potential resilience in determining a cancer prognosis.

This is in line with other studies, which found that people with strong vagal nerve workouts recover more quickly from severe stress by showing much higher levels of inflammatory, cardiovascular and endocrine than people with very low HRV.

A further analysis by an international team of researchers explored the correlation between the vagal overall tone and the survival rates in 87 females suffering from recurrence and metastatic breast cancer.

During a 7-8-year follow-up period, participants with strong HRV earned a median survival rate of 34.9 percent out of 30 7 weeks, whereas persons with poor HRV had a mortality rate of 150 percent. This means that women with a better vagal tone might have higher survival rates than women with poor vagal activity.

The research writers pointed to many possible reasons for this particular result. In the start, higher HRVs could be a symbol for the inflammatory reflex, where the vagus nerve alerts the brain and modulates it by responding to immune systems and neuroendocrine.

Another choice is the fact that greater vagal research is related to social interaction and emotion self-regulation, which may be associated with increased commitment to breast cancer therapy.

Increased vagal activity may also be associated with lower anxiety and increased social support. Recent studies have shown that those with greater vagueness appear to be more pressure resistant, which can be particularly important for the treatment of cancer.

Collectively used, the studies suggest that higher vagal exercise may serve as a defensive component that increases survival latency in prostate, colorectal and breast cancer women and men.

Diabetes Treatment

Diabetes itself refers to several diseases that all alter how your body processes glucose—the primary substance used for energy by your body. Typically, when considering diabetes, you will be looking at two diseases: Type 1 diabetes and type 2 diabetes. These two diseases vary greatly. Women can also develop gestational diabetes as a result of a pregnancy.

These diseases can wreak havoc on the human body, directly influencing how the body functions, heals, and regulates itself. Considering that we primarily eat to raise blood sugar in order to continue functioning at a normal level, having that disconnect and struggle for the body to regulate accordingly can lead to massive issues. The body sometimes struggles to function and heal, and if left untreated without care taken to treat the diseases, it can lead to neuropathy and eventually death. Blood sugar levels that rise too much can cause comas and even death.

The vagus nerve controls the lungs, digestive tract and heart and thus affects the principal functions of breathing, speaking, breathing-opening larynx, sweating, heart beat control, satiety and plundering.

Consequently, the loss of physiologic functions and innervations in the anatomic areas of the body results from diabetic damage to the vagus nerve.

DAN's esophagus disorder affects vagal neuropathy directly. The main effects include heartburn vomiting and difficulties. The reflux is due to the relaxing of the esophagus sphincter, which causes stomach material to back up to the esophagus, causing burning chest pain when feeding, bending, and lying down during the night.

As a diabetic, you may be advised that you are in danger of having one or the terrible health problems this particular disease may cause... Cardiovascular disease... Stroke... Stroke... Renal disorder... Damage to the nerve... Foot and hand neuropathy... Because of glaucoma, retinopathy and cataracts, impaired vision.

You can also deal with severe stomach issues. This is why: the vagus nerve regulates the stomach and intestines muscles. This nerve, which is identical to the other nerves in the body, could be affected if your blood glucose levels are not regulated. This specific disorder is referred to as gastroparesis.

If your vagus nerve is damaged, food flows through your stomach are disrupted, digestion slows down and nutrition is much longer than needed in the body. Probably, the time it takes for food to be digested is unpredictable.

Alzheimer Treatment

Alzheimer's disease sufferers start to see legitimate progress with their cognitive abilities and anxiety related symptoms when they have their vagal nerve stimulated. While it is not entirely known why, it is known that several of the precursor risk factors to Alzheimer's are related to the vagus nerve—high blood pressure can make it more likely that it is developed later in life, which as you know, is linked to the vagus nerve.

More than 4.5 million people are currently impacted by Ad in the United States, and in the absence of preventive measures, it is projected to almost double by 2050.

The acquisition of amyloid plaques and associated neurofibrillary tangles pathologically recognizes advert. Individuals with Alzheimer's (AD) disease have increased tau protein levels of the cerebrospinal fluid (CSF) and decreased amyloid concentrations of CSF.

While individuals with Alzheimer's (AD) disease experience dramatic increases in tau CSF levels which amounts have been shown to be consistent over long periods. Most neurotransmitter mechanisms are modified in AD pathologically. At the start of the disorder, cholinergic neurons in the nucleus basalis of Meynert degenerate.

Such neurons give high projections of link cortices and acetylcholine damage is the mechanical time basis for the inhibition of cholinesterase in the ad remedy.

Furthermore, the glutamatergic activity is dysregulated with inhibition of a pathological stimulation of the NMDA receptor, if the mechanism of the non-competitive antagonist, the Memantine, is systematically clarified.

In contrast to the atrophy of the basal forebrain cholinergic system, the locus coeruleus and raphe nucleus of AD have significant neuronal loss. Significant reductions in the temporal cortex of norepinephrine occur in Ad and correlate with cognitive impairment levels (six).

In animal models, vagus nerve stimulation (VNS) has been found to cause locus ceruleus and to boost the output of norepinephrine into basolateral amygdala and hippocampus.

Additionally, activation of the raphe nucleus with VNS is shown lately.

In the first six months of treatment, Merill et suspected behavioral enhancement results in a small pilot study of ten Ad patients.

They finally published a follow-up study like 7 others, with seventeen patients in no less than one year. Vagus nerve stimulation technique promising brand new impressive alternative approaches, particularly for the treatment of refractory epilepsy in several neurological disorders.

Vagus nerve stimulation technique promising brand new imposing alternative strategies, especially in treating refractory epilepsy in several neurological disorders. In this specific medical research, 14 people with Alzheimer's disease who were treated with VNS were analyzed and the findings were analyzed in the literature glow.

The research covered only the first and second phase of Ad patients. A total of 14 advertisements (seven males and seven female adults aged 68 to 82 years old) participated in this study. For one season, patients are followed up.

Once each implant has been activated (two days after implantation), individuals ' engagement has been significantly increased, and continues to improve.

Usually, it appears after age 60, but it is possible for younger people to suffer from the disease as well. It is not considered normal, nor to be expected through aging. What it does, however, is disrupt daily life and can require the individual suffering from it to require long-term or around-the-clock care by licensed medical professionals.

There is currently evidence that high blood pressure and cholesterol may be responsible for raising the chances for ever developing the disease, and that certain activities, such as socializing, exercising the brain, and physically exercising yourself can lessen the risk.

The use of vagus nerve stimulation is being researched as a possible treatment for Alzheimer's disease, showing that there are changes in quality of life for those who are treated with the stimulation.

Autism Treatment

New research in vagal stimulation and toning is giving those with autism hope. Autism is a diverse condition that affects individuals uniquely. Many are diagnosed with the disorder at a very young age and is a condition that stays with them for their whole life. Some symptoms of autism may lesson as children and parents are given many new opportunities to help cope and manage symptoms with early intervention strategies.

Since the vagus nerve directly affects heart rate and when weakened makes it more difficult for the parasympathetic system to maintain control some behaviors and symptoms may be triggered or a result of a dysfunctional vagus nerve. Because of their diagnosis, children tend to reside in flight or fight mode, which is what commonly causes meltdowns. Being able to easily transition out of fight or flight mode is made more difficult for ASD children because of the sensory processing issues.

Incorporating regular exercises that address the sensory needs and challenges for children on the spectrum can help with multiply processing disorders. Some of the best activities and exercises for children on the spectrum include:

1. **Therapeutic Listening.** Therapeutic listening is a complex form of listening therapy that includes the entire audio sensory system. This form of listening, however, goes beyond just the audio senses; it helps develop a child's active listening skills that are necessary for communication. Since the vagus nerve connects to the inner ear, this form of therapy can also have an impact on other sensory development and can help a child have better control over their behavioral actions. Therapeutic listening uses specially designed sounds and music to activate all levels of the audio system. It helps highlight noise that will allow the child to hone in on one noise while being able to dull out the rest of the sounds. This requires the use of headphones to accompany the music, which brings balance to the song. The music or sounds vary and can be intentionally chosen to help a

child work on their own specific needs. The convenient aspect of therapeutic listening is that it does not require having to follow a detailed plan. The types of music chosen can be switched if the needs of the child are not being met. Unlike many other therapy programs that require create goals and action plans at the start of the session, therapeutic listening depends on how the child reacts to the music. If certain sounds seem to overstimulate or under-stimulate the child, the music is reevaluated and a new set of songs or music is chosen. The music also uniquely allows the child to bring awareness to their body movement. For many children, the music will initiate a swaying movement that aligns with the rhyme of the song being listened to. It should be done for no more than 30 minutes twice a day, allowing for four hours to pass between each session. You can see instant results where your child may move with more precision, focus more, and their body will be more calm and relaxed. Long-term benefits can allow children to focus in school, make meaningful connections, and live a more functional life. Therapeutic listening effectively stimulates the vagus nerve and encourages the activation of the rest and relax response. Children can learn to navigate out of their fight or flight response and come to a place where they feel safe and secure.

2. **Humming**. The vagus nerve contributes to many elements of the vocal system, which also connects the inner ear. When humming, the vibrations stimulate the vagus nerve both through its connection with the vocal cords and the ear. These vibrations can create a calming and soothing sensation for those with spectrum disorder. Humming is also a way that individuals can bring balance to the vestibular system and may help them feel more steady and in control.

3. **Movements**. Children with spectrum disorder tend to exhibit unusual behavior. One common behavior of children on the spectrum is rocking or swinging. You can often observe children seeking out specific movements of this manner. This is often due to the attempt to self regulate and stimulate the vagus nerve. They also tend to make repetitive movements that can resemble a mild case of obsessive-compulsive disorder. These unusual movements and repetitive actions are actually ways children unintentionally activate their vagus nerve. Some of these movements include: Spinning, Climbing, Hand flapping, Rocking, Humming, Throwing things, Biting or chewing, Aggressively grabbing and squeezing items.

You can help your child find the most effective movement by honing in on which of these movements tends to have the most calming and soothing effect on them.

Migraine Treatment

Migraine, a neurologically very impaired disease, is characterized by frequent, moderate to severe impacts associated with vegetative symptoms. Patients with regular attacks could overuse medications, leading to overuse of headache and chronic migraine.

Neuromodulatory methods have been developed over the past decade because of the management of headaches that do not respond correctly to treatment.

Invasive hypothalamic, supraorbital, and occipital Neurostimulation, sphenopalatine ganglia and atriotemporal nerves generated promising results. Invasive procedure, Vagus nerve stimulation (VNS) is suitable for clinically refractive depression and epilepsy. In intractable migraine with comorbid anxiety, this has a clinical benefit.

Experimentally, VNS has modulated neurotransmitters, affected cerebral blood and metabolism in limbic system and pain matrix areas, as well as had inflammatory and acidic pain impact.

The proposed VNS elements on soreness routes that include the modulation of the amount of extra glutamate in the caudal trigeminal nucleus, pain management outcomes and the modulation of cortical excitability.

Article hoc test information leads to a good literature on vagus nerve stimulation by steadily and rapidly decreasing the therapy severity of pain and by reducing the use of recovery medication by people with episodic migraine.

The effectiveness and protection of noninvasive vagus nerve stimulation (nVNS) in people with migraine have been demonstrated. Outcomes of the NVNS prospective study for the Acute Migraine Treatment (PRESTO) study found that therapy with self-administered devices for the vast majority of endpoints–like pain tolerance, pain relief, and multi-time respondent prices above 50 percent–is much better than fake.

Results of the article hoc analysis now add to the beneficial literature and conclude the procedure reliably and rapidly increasing pain severity while reducing the intake of rehabilitation medicine.

Between January 11, 2016 and March 130, 2017 the PRESTO study consisted of 285 individuals with an episodic migraine from ten websites and included three periods, each lasting for four weeks: a span in which people were given their regular drugs, a double blind time in which patients are provided randomly, sometimes by NVNS or fake care, and an open label duration.

Up to five migraine strikes are advised to be healed over the double-blind duration and up to five more VNS attacks throughout the open mark period. Within 20 minutes of the onset of migraine pain, people administered the unit themselves.

The findings of the analysis showed that, in the first procedure, the proportion of individuals that obtained a minimum of 1-point decline in severity was significantly higher for the nVNS cohort than in the placebo collection from 30 minutes (32.2% versus 18.5%), sixty minutes (38.8% versus 24.0%), and 120 minutes (46.8% versus 26.2%).

For these hits, there have been more improvements to the nVNS cohort by one point or more than 60 minutes (33.3 percent vs. 22.2 percent) and 120 (39.4 percent vs. 26.4 percent) for the bogus cohort.

Likewise, for the first strike (59.3 percent versus 41.9 percent) and those attacks (52.3 versus 37.3 percent), the proportion of individuals who did not operate on rescue care was significantly higher.

For people who started therapy, the differences for painless prices between nVNS and shame were far more pronounced, when the strike was mild, than people who waited until the pain was serious or moderate to treat their attack, the researchers addressed.

The number of individuals who effectively aborted a gentle first migraine experience was significantly higher with nVNS than with the bugger from 120 minutes (50% vs 25%).

Based on the information, scientists argue that the treatment can be an efficient, viable option for people to relieve pain without increasing exposure to adverse pharmacological events or drug overuse.

Epilepsy Treatment

Epilepsy is another common chronic disorder that people around the world suffer from. When someone suffers from epilepsy, they suffer from abnormal brain activity. This can cause periods of time in which they suffer from seizures or loss of consciousness. It is something that happens around the world, to people of all ages and backgrounds.

Epilepsy itself is a seizure disorder—it can vary greatly from person to person, but what is consistent is that the individual has abnormal brain activity. Seizures themselves can vary, and typically, those who have been diagnosed with epilepsy must have had at least two seizures that are confirmed before the diagnosis is given in the first place.

For some people, epilepsy can be treated with medication. For others, surgery can help manage the symptoms. Some people will age out of the seizures while others may suffer all their lives. Due to the complexity and variability of the brain, epilepsy does not present the same way in every person out there—it will vary based on the individual. That does not necessarily change the diagnosis—it just means that the treatment plan may vary.

Vagus nerve stimulation (VNS) involves sending a message to the brain through the use of an surgically implanted small medical device through sometimes gentle electrical stimulation from the vagus nerve in the chest. No brain surgery is needed.

This pulse or stimulation is provided in the same way as a pacemaker by a medical unit. The vagus nerve is an autonomous nervous system component that regulates the body's involuntary function.

VNS may be able to manage epilepsy in cases where antiepileptic drugs are ineffective or have intolerable side effects. VNS works well to stop seizures in some patients.

The implanted health-related device is a sluggish, round electric battery and measures on the silver dollar dimensions. Cyberonics, Inc. developed the VNS medical device.

The doctor decides the power and timing of the unit's pulses, based on the individual needs of each patient. With no additional operation, the degree of electric stimulation could be converted and a programming wall connected to a notebook computer.

Unwanted side effects of VNS may include hoaxing, vomiting, a sore throat, shortness of breath, a very short feeling of coughing, altered vocal tone, tooth pain, ear pain, and a tingling sensation in the chest. Skin irritation or infection can occur on the website of the implantation. VNS does not affect the human brain negatively.

This is a major operation and should not be taken lightly. It can be the last choice for all people with unrestricted epileptic seizures. Consider all options until seizure control is offered. Stimulation of the nerve is a mechanism used to regulate epileptic seizures. It requires the use of a small unit on the dimensions of a silver dollar which directs moderate electrical impulses to the brain through a nerve known as the vagus nerve in the neck.

To insert the device, a small incision is made in the neck together with a small incision below the collarbone. When the battery is working, an electric pulse generator is installed, a flexible disconnected plastic tube is powered with electrodes under your skin to the left neck vagus.

The generator delivers 30 second pulses of energy every 5 minutes to the vagus nerve. Those stimuli block the disturbances of energy in the human brain.

Doctors and scientists are not yet sure how epilepsy and the vagus nerve are intricately related. What is known, however, is that shocking or stimulating the vagus nerve is an effective way to end a seizure in progress. Scientists noticed this connection in the 19th century, when they realized that sometimes, seizures would stop when pressure was applied to the carotid artery. As you may remember, the carotid artery and vagus nerve go together for a short period of time in the neck.

Over time, it was found that stimulating the nerve with electrical impulses would show a decrease in seizures in general. It is not necessarily immediate, but over time, through stimulation, the seizure activity slowed, and some people saw a cessation in seizures altogether.

When you are using vagus nerve stimulation to treat your epilepsy, you will have a small device implanted near your collarbone. It is then programmed to stimulate your vagus nerve at regular intervals, while also programmed to create a sudden burst of stimulation, which can be done with the use of a magnet to interrupt a seizure that is in progress at any given moment.

Despite the fact that scientists do not yet understand this link, it is undeniable—it does work to lessen seizure activity. Within a few months, around ¼ of people see that their seizure frequency has dropped in half. And after a year or two, upwards of 45% of people have found that the frequency of epileptic episodes has dropped by half. Of course, this treatment should never be taken instead of medication that has been prescribed by a doctor.

Sleeping Disorder Treatment

Your body needs sleep to function, and a massive portion of your life will be spent slept away.

Nevertheless, the effects of sleep deprivation are incredibly real and noticeable after a relatively short period of time. It takes only about 20 hours before the body starts to show noticeable signs of sleep deprivation. Before we continue on with this chapter, however, let's stop and take a look at what sleep actually is in the first place.

Obstructive sleeping disorder is where there's a blockage in the upper aviation routes. This outcome in stops in breathing for the duration of the night that may make you suddenly wake up, regularly with a gagging sound. Wheezing generally happens in this issue.

Anxious legs disorder may likewise trigger dozing trouble. This condition creates awkward uproars in your legs, for example, shivering or hurting. These sensations give you the desire to make your legs move now and again, including while at the same time resting, which can interfere with your rest.

Postponed rest stage issue is another condition that can influence rest. This condition causes a postponement in the 24-hour cycle of rest and attentiveness. You may not feel tired or nod off until the center of the night. This rest cycle makes it harder for you to get up in the early morning and prompts daytime weariness.

Due to the heightened sympathetic response when the parasympathetic responses are muted, the individual will find themselves struggling to sleep well, all because the nerve that is supposed to regulate their ability to sleep fails to regulate itself.

Sleep disorders vary from type to type, but there are several that exist. This particular section will look at sleep disorders that are believed to be related, at least in some way, to the vagus nerve. These all share similar symptoms—you will likely be sleepy during the day and may struggle to fall asleep or stay asleep at night. Some people will also go on to fall asleep during times that are considered dangerous or inappropriate, such as at work or even when driving a car.

- Insomnia: When you suffer from insomnia, you usually either struggle to sleep at night or you cannot stay asleep at night. You may find yourself regularly waking up, despite your best efforts to clean up your sleep hygiene.

- Sleep apnea: When you suffer from sleep apnea, your breathing patterns when asleep are abnormal. This can be due to some sort of neurological issue, or also because you have slept in a strange position or are obese and have an obstruction of your windpipe when in lying down positions. This is something that most people do not notice when they are sleeping, but the impacts can be extreme. This can result in heart damage or death if left untreated.
- Restless legs syndrome: When you suffer from RLS, you have a sleep movement disorder. This causes you to feel like your legs are uncomfortable when you try to sleep, leading to you feeling the urge to move while attempting to fall asleep. In some cases, this can wake you up in the middle of the night as well, leading to struggles in staying asleep.
- Narcolepsy: When you suffer from narcolepsy, you feel extremely sleepy during the day and may even fall asleep at inopportune times suddenly and unexpectedly during the night. These people struggle to regulate their sleep-wake cycles, which leads to them feeling rested right after they wake up, but feeling sleepy throughout much of the day. Their sleep cycles are usually disjointed and not particularly restful.

Rest trouble may influence your physical and emotional wellness. Absence of rest may likewise make you have visit migraines or issues focusing. The vast majority experience trouble resting sooner or later in their lives. A few people may feel revived after just six or seven hours of rest. In any case, most grownups need around eight hours of rest each night to feel rested. Indications of dozing trouble may incorporate powerlessness to center during the day, visit migraines, fractiousness, daytime weakness, getting up too soon, awakening for the duration of the night, or taking a few hours to nod off. You may likewise experience low vitality during the day or have recognizably dark circles under your eyes. Sleeping disorder can be a nuisance and cause physical and mental tiredness.

It has been found that the vagus nerve stimulator, in particular the electrical stimulator, can cause an increase in apnea. This apnea can also worsen the occurrence rate of seizures in general, making it difficult to determine whether stimulating the vagus nerve electrically is a good fit for those struggling with sleep apnea or other sleep disorders, so it is advisable to use exercise and other methods to stimulate your vagus nerve.

Trauma And Ptsd Treatment

Trauma is something everyone experiences at some point in their lives. While it can be overcome, trauma can have a long-lasting impact on an individual, causing distress diminishing self-worth, and causing a wide range of psychological concerns. On top of the psychological effects, trauma can greatly impair an individual's physical health due to its side effects.

Trauma occurs as a natural response from the body trying to cope and manage overwhelming, disturbing, and stressful situations or events. Trauma can cause an individual to feel hopeless, depressed, and significant distrust.

PTSD can arise out of traumatic occurrences. Those with PTSD tend to have symptoms of trauma and/or acute stress disorder but the symptoms never diminish and can last for months or longer. The longer the symptoms are present, the more debilitating and severe they become.

They can act out aggressively and abusively exhibit behavior that can be viewed as detached or erratic. The symptoms tend to be grouped into four categories, but the severity of the symptoms can range greatly.

When individuals are faced with constant trauma, they are unable to allow the parasympathetic nervous system to become active and the vagus nerve reduces the fight or flight response. They often enter into a state of constant shutdown where they feel they are not living their own life. This leads to confusion and the inability to recognize a safe situation, places, or people. Those who suffer from PTSD can suffer more severely from this as they are more likely to replay the traumatic events repeatingly through their minds. When they continuously loop these memories, it makes it more difficult for them to distinguish between what is real and what is just a recollection of past events. In order for individuals to learn to cope with their trauma, they need to be able to break this negative loop.

The occurrences of mischievous memories may include: sporadic, unwelcome disturbing memories of the terrible mishap, remembering the horrible accident as if it were occurring again (flashbacks), Disquieting hallucinations or bad dreams about the horrific mishap, Extreme passionate difficulty, or physical reactions to something that makes you remember the horrific incident that happened.

Stay away from places, experiences, and people who help you to recall this awful tragedy, Negative developments in perception and mental state. The side effects of negative changes in intuition or mental condition may be depressive feelings regarding yourself, other people or the universe, Sadness about what is to come and memory issues.

Constraint to preserve warm relations, feeling limited to family and friends, absence of workout excitement you once enjoyed, having problem with keeping positive feelings, and also feeling a state of numbness.

Breathing plays a major part in overcoming trauma. Those with PTSD frequently suffer from panic or anxiety attacks. This causes their breathing to be rapid and focused in the upper chest. When you see an animal face a predator, they will often freeze and/or play dead. While this is effective for in the wild when facing down a lion, for humans this response is a hindrance and not the way many want to live out their days. Being able to notice and regain control over your breathing can help the vagus nerve and parasympathetic system click on.

While it can take a great deal of practice being able to put a sudden stop to the shutdown response, gaining control of your breathing and working through your trauma instead of avoiding it can be done. With vagus nerve stimulation and toning, individuals can retrain their systems to react in a more appropriate manner when facing trauma. Even those with severe PTSD can benefit from learning how to perform quick vagus nerve activation techniques to help work through traumatic episodes. Through vagus nerve stimulation, those suffering through trauma and/or PTSD can rewire their process and become unstuck from the fight or flight, or shutdown, phases.

Stimulating the vagus to stop the sympathetic system is done when the individuals feels safe and secure. The following activities can instantly promote varying levels of these feelings.

Hug. Along with the first technique, hugging helps us feel safe and connected to others. By giving or receiving a hug, you can instantly trigger the vagus nerve.

- Laugh. If hugging is not really your thing, you can laugh instead. Laughing can help stimulate the vagus nerve to release oxytocin. Oxytocin encourages you to make connections with others and lift your mood. Laughing, just like hugging, helps you feel connected with others and can strengthen bonds.

- Shake it off. One of the ways you can bounce out of the shutdown mode is to do a full body shake. Before you go into a full out shake, do a quick body scan. Are there any areas of your body that feel tense or stiff? If you find tension in your body, these are the areas you want to focus on when you wiggle and shake. Give each area your attention as you shake the tension out. When you have gone through all the areas and feel relieved, pause for a moment to take in the stillness that surrounds you and let it fill you. This is your body waking up again. This is the feeling you want to recall when facing a trauma-induced memory or episode.

Healing from trauma or PTSD can be a lifelong process. Strengthening the vagus nerve daily results in developing the skills necessary for your mind and body to bounce back from traumatic events and experiences that trigger trauma symptoms. Keep in mind just how intricately linked to fight-flight-freeze and rest-and-digest the vagus nerve is and consider for a moment what PTSD is. It involves regulating the fear response, as well as telling the body when that fear response is appropriate. If PTSD is largely due to an inability to regulate those responses to the trauma, it stands to reason that the two are intricately linked to each other.

Evidence has shown that those suffering from PTSD do, in fact, show a diminished functioning of the parasympathetic nervous system, implying that it is not regulating itself effectively and because the body is never able to put the individual into rest-and-digest mode due to the lack of the parasympathetic activity triggering the proper hormones, instead the individual is stuck in fight-flight-freeze mode. Consider the symptoms for a moment: Feeling guarded and afraid are two major symptoms of PTSD, and both of them are directly related to the sympathetic nervous system being in control. Now consider insomnia, which is an inability to sleep. That inability to sleep is related to the fact that the body cannot get itself out of fight-flight-freeze mode. During that time, the individual is stuck awake, no matter how tired he or she may be feeling, all because the body is unable to relax enough to effectively sleep.

When the parasympathetic nervous system takes control defensively, as is common in PTSD, the body shuts down on itself. It overcorrects, leading to a numbness or freeze response. Then, with people with PTSD, they are reacting with an overactive or underactive vagus nerve, leading to that feeling of shutting down and being numb or unable to feel joy.

Rheumatoid Arthritis Treatment

Rheumatoid arthritis is a disorder that falls into two different classifications that you have already seen thus far—it is an inflammatory autoimmune disorder. Remember, inflammatory disorders cause inflammation in the area, and the autoimmune disorder then attacks that particular area.

While some arthritis, namely osteoarthritis, is caused through simple wear-and-tear that is caused through overuse, rheumatoid arthritis is entirely self-inflicted—just not consciously. You cannot control that your body is attacking itself, and yet it continues to do so, sending the immune system after your joints or other body parts and attacking them. The lining in your joints can become weakened and painful, and you may even start to damage bone.

Rheumatoid arthritis can be broken down into two key words: Rheumatoid and arthritis. This offers you plenty of insight into what it is. Rheumatoid itself refers to inflammation or pain, particularly where it lingers in any sorts of joints or muscles. Arthritis itself refers to any sort of joint inflammation. This makes rheumatoid arthritis almost redundant, but there is a reason for that—it is joint inflammation and pain that is literally caused by inflammation. The autoantibodies created by virtue of having an autoimmune disorder attack and inflame the joints, which then leads to arthritis to develop.

It is particularly notable because it is largely symmetrical—it will occur on both sides of the body at the same time rather than developing due to wear on specific joints. However, rheumatoid arthritis does not stop at your joints: It can also impact the rest of your body—even in areas where there are no bones at all, such as the heart or lungs.

Rheumatoid arthritis has warning signs and symptoms that can cue you to making a point to investigate whatever is happening to you at that particular moment. When you suffer from rheumatoid arthritis, it may be easy to try to brush the pain off as being indicative of your aging, but remember, it is not a normal side effect of aging. Sure, you will feel slower and stiffer, but you should not have all of the inflammation and angry, red joints that go along with rheumatoid arthritis to begin with. Let's stop and take a look at the most common rheumatoid arthritis symptoms: Joint pain, stiffness, and fatigue.

Joint pain is usually characterized as either being slow-going or sudden in onset, depending on the individual. The individual will likely find that they have swollen joints that may look inflamed and red, meaning they are warm to the touch and also noticeably different. These joints can eventually disfigure if left untreated. The stiffness typically occurs first thing in the morning, or after a period of time in which you sat without moving for a while, such as if you work at a desk. You will feel stiff, and in some instances, like you cannot move at all. Fatigue is relatively straightforward—when you suffer from rheumatoid arthritis, you have a tendency to be exhausted sooner and longer than other people.

Rheumatoid arthritis has warning signs and symptoms that can cue you to making a point to investigate whatever is happening to you at that particular moment. When you suffer from rheumatoid arthritis, it may be easy to try to brush the pain off as being indicative of your aging, but remember, it is not a normal side effect of aging. Sure, you will feel slower and stiffer, but you should not have all of the inflammation and angry, red joints that go along with rheumatoid arthritis to begin with. Let's stop and take a look at the most common rheumatoid arthritis symptoms: Joint pain, stiffness, and fatigue.

Joint pain is usually characterized as either being slow-going or sudden in onset, depending on the individual. The individual will likely find that they have swollen joints that may look inflamed and red, meaning they are warm to the touch and also noticeably different. These joints can eventually disfigure if left untreated. The stiffness typically occurs first thing in the morning, or after a period of time in which you sat without moving for a while, such as if you work at a desk. You will feel stiff, and in some instances, like you cannot move at all. Fatigue is relatively straightforward—when you suffer from rheumatoid arthritis, you have a tendency to be exhausted sooner and longer than other people.

By now, you should be pretty confident in your understanding of the link between the vagus nerve and inflammation and autoimmune disease. We have already established that the vagus nerve is responsible for sending the signals necessary to the brain to allow for the regulation of the immune system, which, when overstimulated or under-stimulated, can lead to a misfiring of the immune system, which can be particularly problematic for the individual suffering. This can cause either an immune system that is not functioning at all, or one that functions too well and attacks the body instead.

When you wish to treat your rheumatoid arthritis, then, you want to stimulate the vagus nerve, causing an inhibition of cytokine production, which should also reduce the inflammation associated with rheumatoid arthritis in the first place. There has been success using vagus nerve stimulators to create electrical impulses that travel directly to the vagus nerve, which then influences how the body is regulated. Those with rheumatoid arthritis who have attempted treatment in these manners have found that they show a massive improvement in their symptoms—they showed significant reduction in their DAS28-CRP scores, which is the measure of how active rheumatoid arthritis is at any given moment. Those pre-treatments were shown to have a 4.19, and after a week, they saw this number reduced down to 3.12, which shows mild activation of the disease at any given moment.

Effectively, then, you can use a vagus nerve stimulator to lessen the severity of your arthritis thanks to the anti-inflammatory effect of the stimulation in the first place. That reduction in symptoms can be significant, allowing for a massive improvement in quality of life that can be the difference between enjoying day-to-day activities and being entirely miserable in the first place.

Conclusion

The vagus nerve is something more people need to talk about and understand. Knowing and understanding what your vagus nerve is good for can help others rectify various health conditions. Most don't even realize the power of their vagus nerve, and how a vagus nerve that isn't in-tune with the rest of the body can adversely affect it.

Constant illness and disease can have a huge impact on our quality of life. When we are constantly unwell both physically and psychologically, our productivity, ability to engage with others, and capacity for stress management are all greatly diminished. Accessing the power of the vagus nerve through stimulation gives you back the power to take charge of your health and ensure that your body is functioning at its best.

When we fully understand the power of the Vagus nerve and the significance of its parasympathetic responses in the body, we can then begin to unleash the ability of the body to heal itself and use this as a way of boosting our immunity, enhancing our cognitive abilities, and improving our emotional health.

By understanding this nerve, the mind-body connection, and the body's natural response systems, individuals who suffer from mental distress and physical health conditions can learn to take control of their well-being.

Now that you have been armed with the world's greatest secrets to unlocking your body's new potential, what will you do with them? It is now time to start your healing process, no matter what ailment you may be experiencing. Use the power of the vagus nerve to unlock your beauty and power within, reduce your stress levels, and find the ultimate level of calm within yourself!

Your vagus nerve is small, but it's incredibly powerful, and if you're not taking care of it, problems can arise. Take the time to focus on improving your vagal tone and stimulating your vagus nerve. The vagus nerve could change your life. Knowing its functions and how you can stimulate can lead you to a more fulfilled, more aware, and happy life.

The vagus nerve is a part of you. Understand and master your own personal control over it, and see its effects come to life.

CPSIA information can be obtained
at www.ICGtesting.com
Printed in the USA
LVHW051037260121
677404LV00007B/352

9 781914 193507